Goiter - Causes and Treatment

Edited by N.K. Agrawal

Published in London, United Kingdom

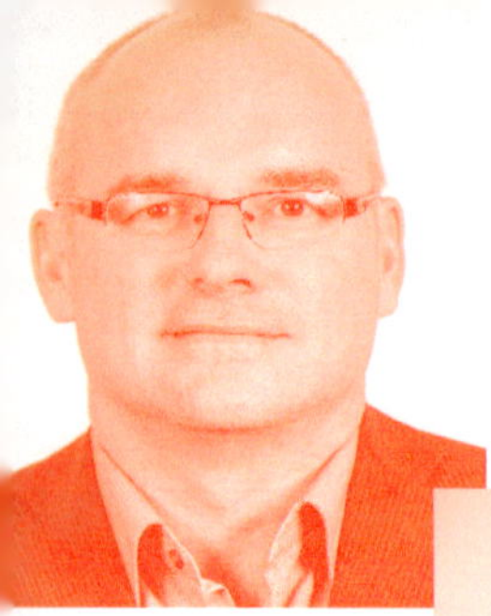
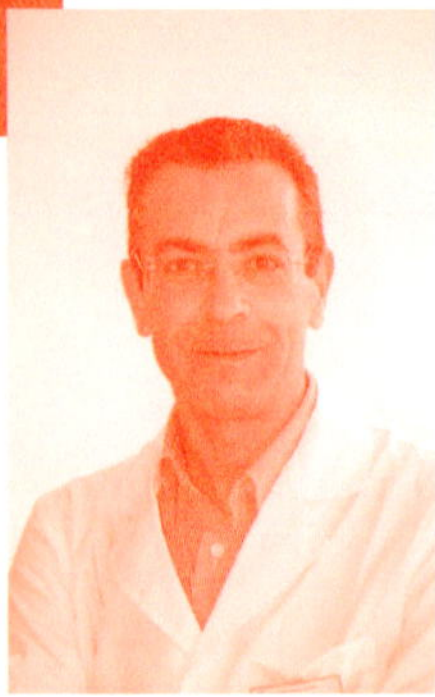
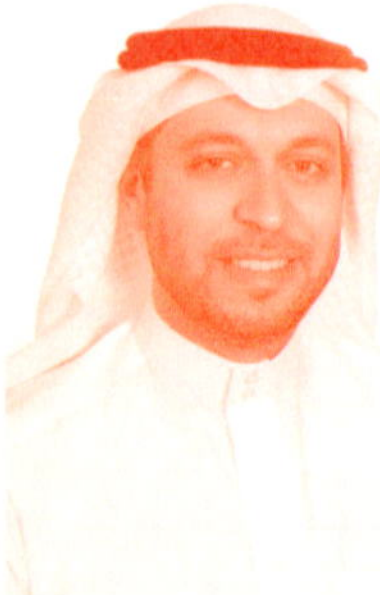
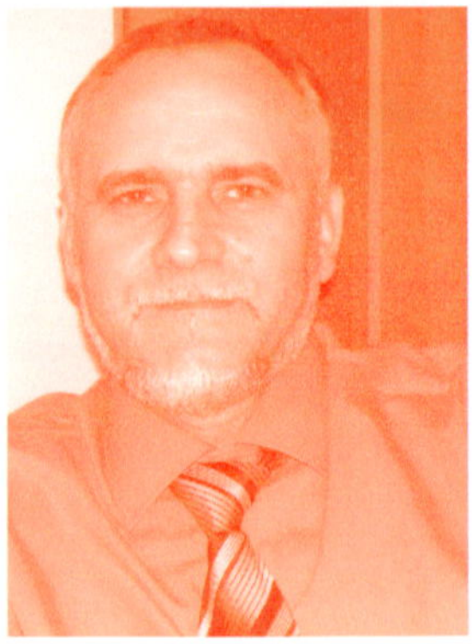
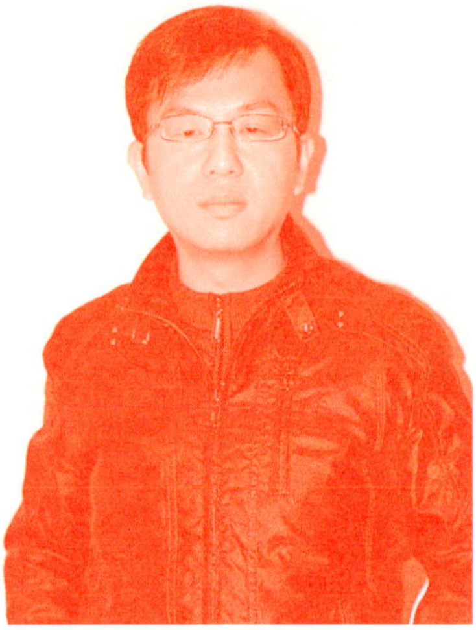
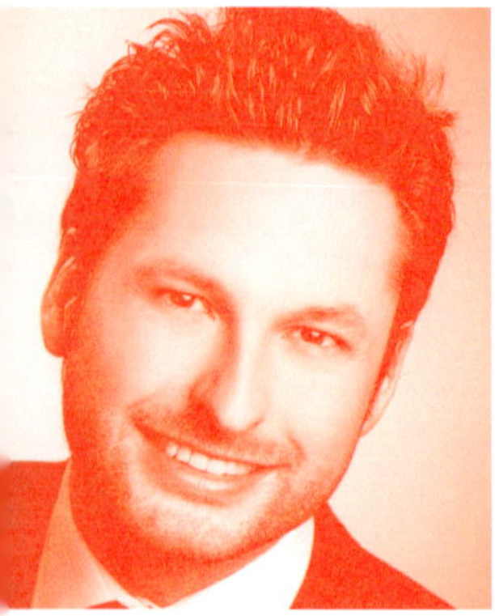
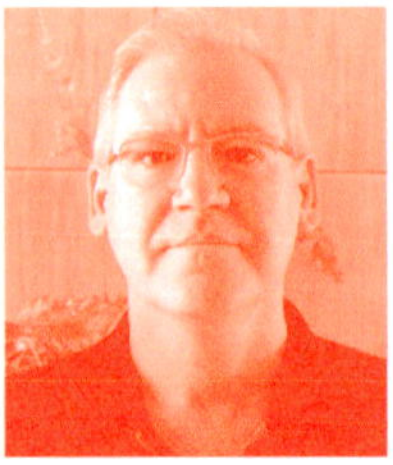

IntechOpen

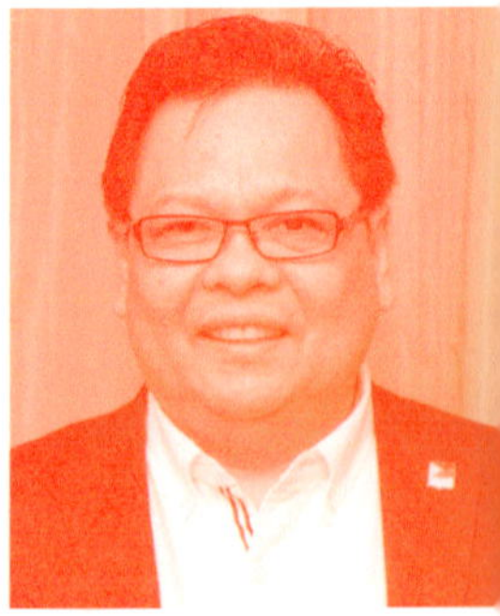
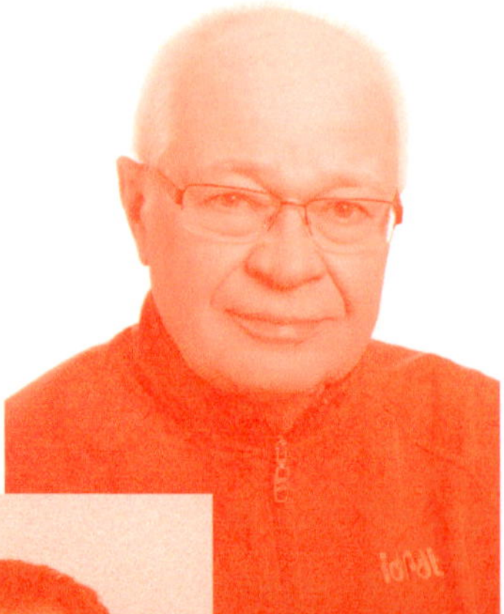
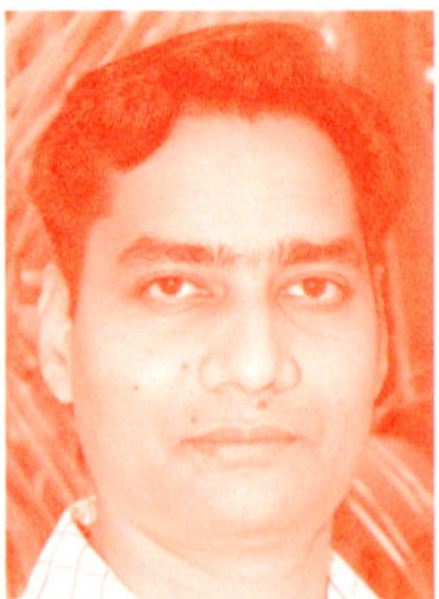
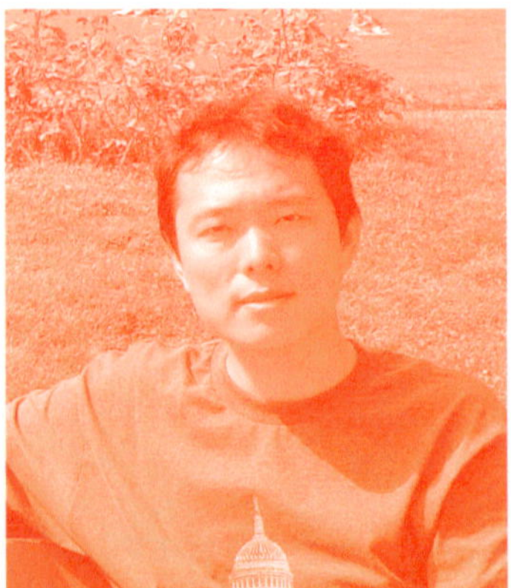
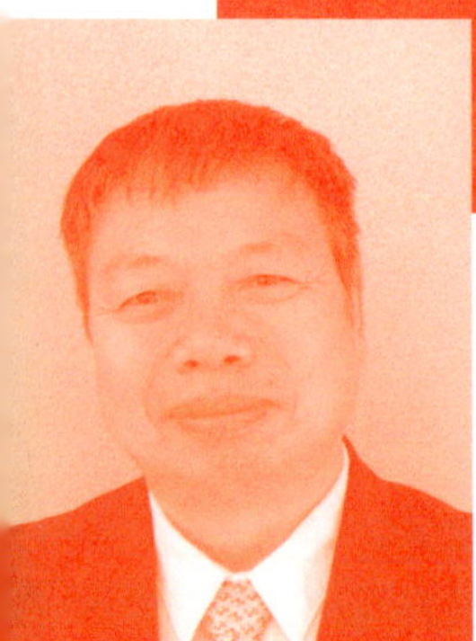
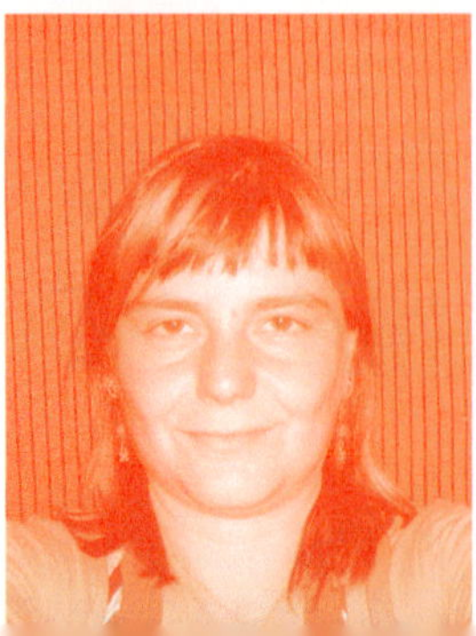

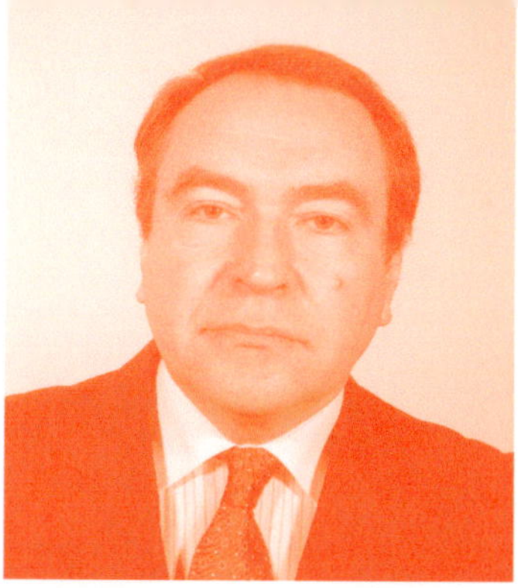

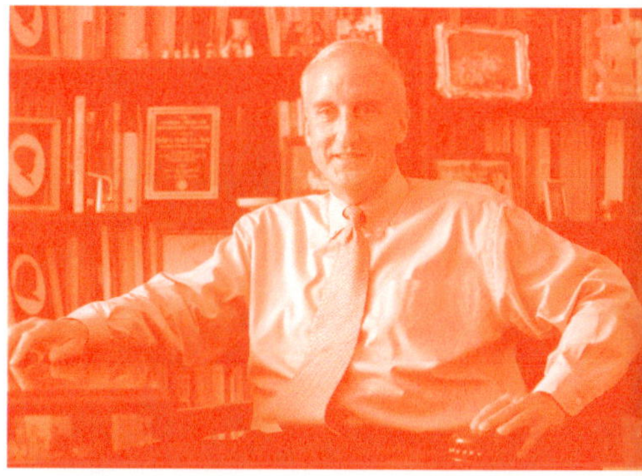

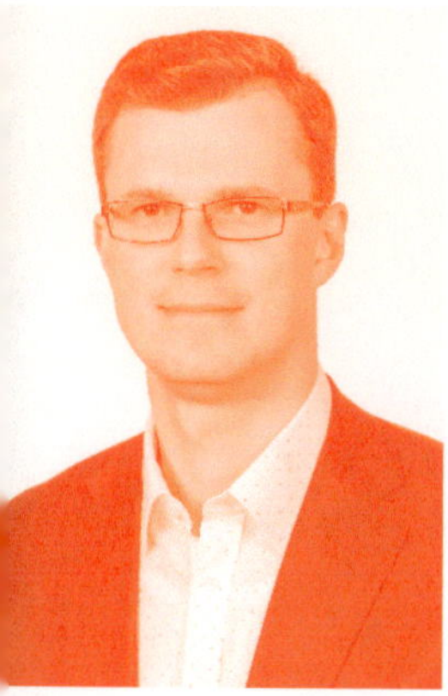

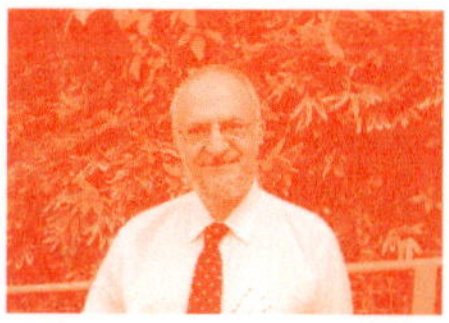

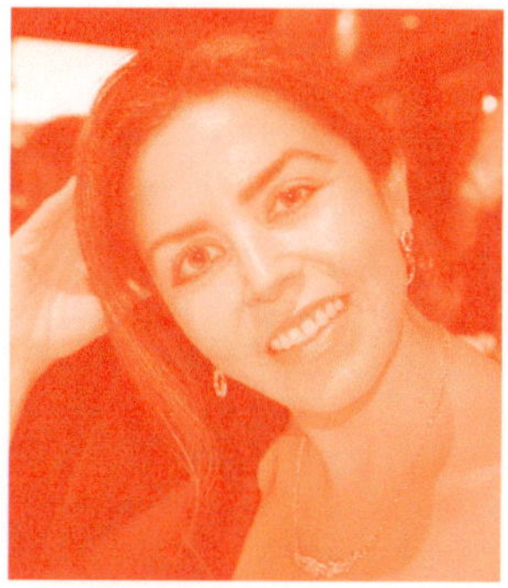

Supporting open minds since 2005

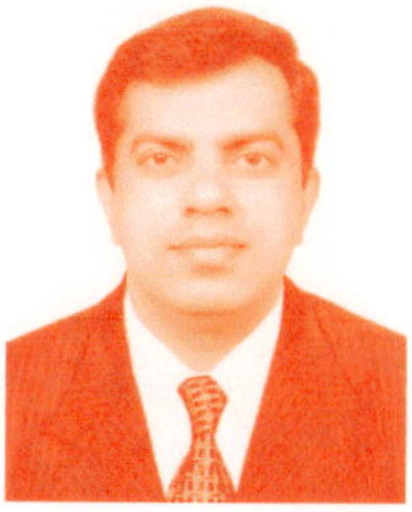

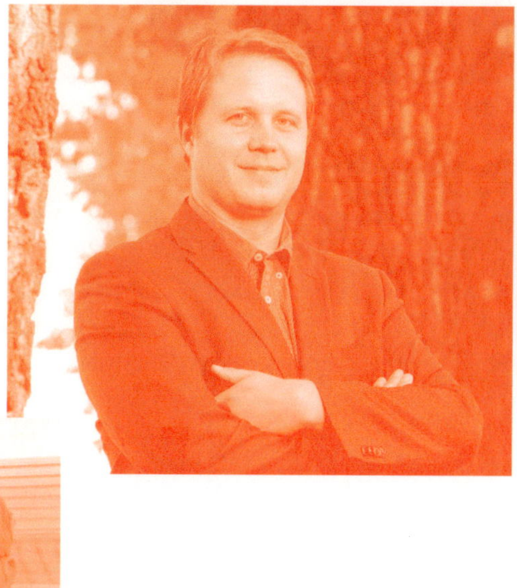

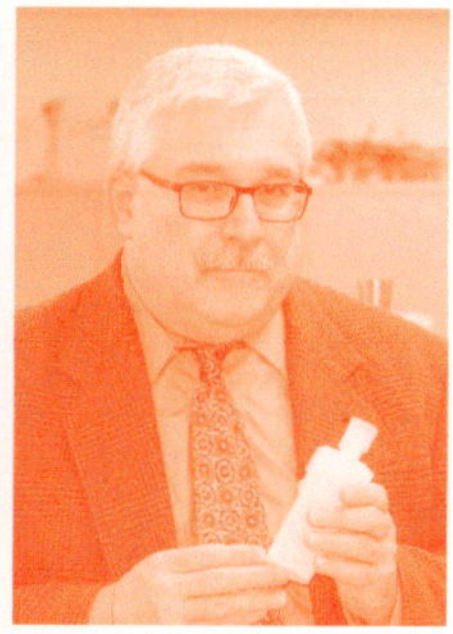

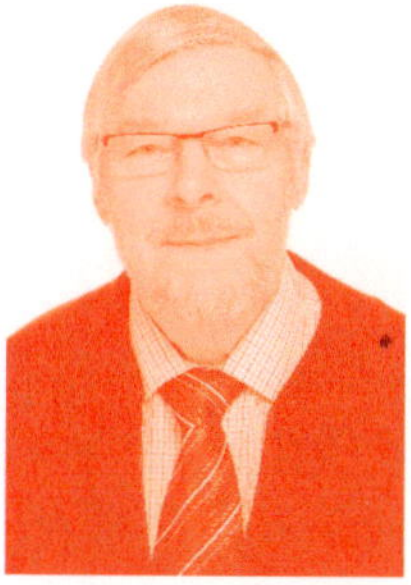

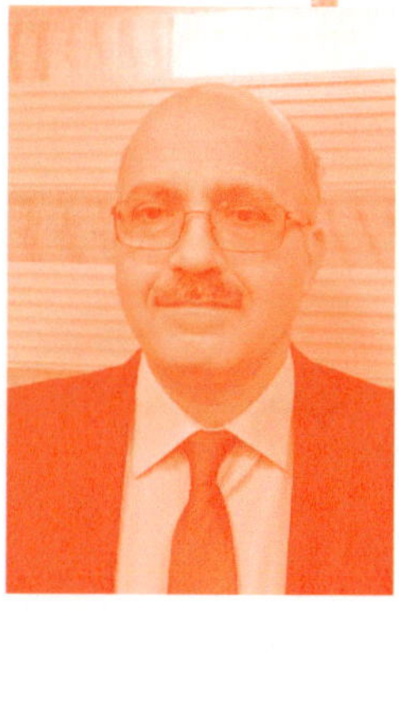

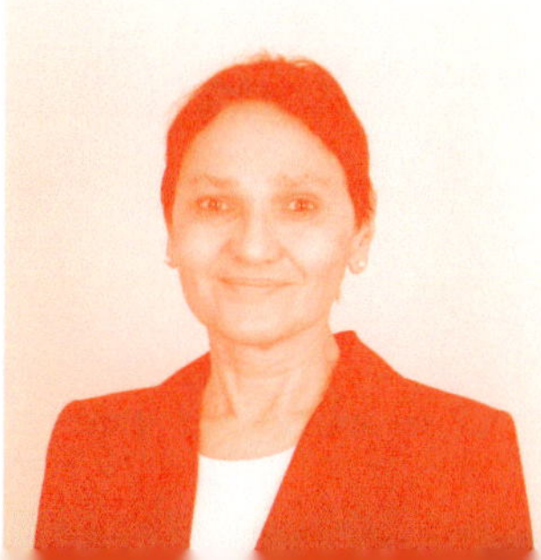

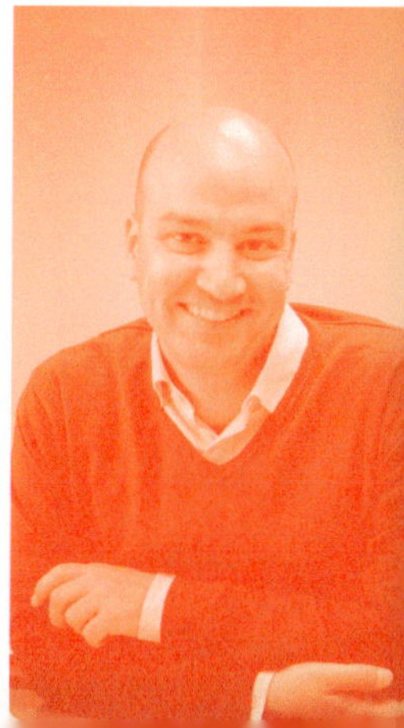

Goiter - Causes and Treatment
http://dx.doi.org/10.5772/intechopen.83073
Edited by N.K. Agrawal

Contributors
Prakruti Dash, Rajlaxmi Tiwari, Balamurugan Pandiyan, Madhukar Mittal, Vanishri Ganakumar, Ravindra Shukla, Mk Garg, Rushikesh Maheshwari, N.K. Agrawal, Dhananjay Ms, Piyush Gupta, Sanjay Saran, Melinda Kolcsar, Zsolt Gáll, Rahul Pandey, Sanjeev Kumar, Narendra Kotwal

First published in London, United Kingdom, 2020 by IntechOpen
IntechOpen is the global imprint of INTECHOPEN LIMITED, registered in England and Wales, registration number: 11086078, 7th floor, 10 Lower Thames Street, London, EC3R 6AF, United Kingdom
Printed in Croatia

British Library Cataloguing-in-Publication Data
A catalogue record for this book is available from the British Library

Additional hard and PDF copies can be obtained from orders@intechopen.com

Goiter - Causes and Treatment
Edited by N.K. Agrawal
p. cm.
Print ISBN 978-1-78985-963-8
Online ISBN 978-1-78985-964-5
eBook (PDF) ISBN 978-1-78985-872-3

For EU product safety concerns:
IN TECH d.o.o., Prolaz Marije Krucifikse Kozulić 3, 51000 Rijeka, Croatia, info@intechopen.com or visit our website at intechopen.com.

Meet the editor

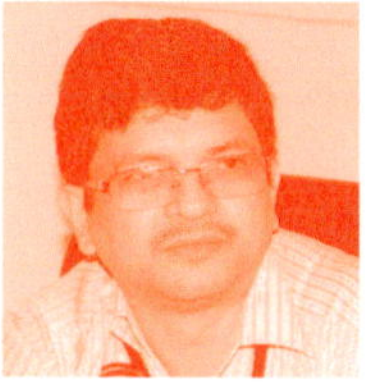

Prof. Neeraj Kumar Agrawal, DM (Endocrinology) is a Professor in the Department of Endocrinology and Metabolism, Institute of Medical Sciences, Banaras Hindu University, Varanasi, India. He has clinical and research training in endocrinology and metabolism. He completed his DM course (Endocrinology) (post-doctoral) in 2000 and since then has been actively involved in teaching and training in the subspeciality. He has keen interest in reproductive endocrinology and adolescent endocrinology, diabetes, and thyroid disorders. He has published over 95 scientific publications in peer-reviewed journals and conference proceedings. He has edited a book on "Thyroid Hormone" and "Debatable Topics in PCOS Patients". He is an examiner to training centres of endocrinology. He is actively involved in the Endocrine Society of India and is a speaker in annual conferences.

Contents

Preface

Thyroid gland disorders are common worldwide. Of the diseases affecting the thyroid gland, enlargement of this gland appears to be very intriguing and perplexing. The gland may be diffusely affected or may be focally involved. There is a need for updated concise information from experts. The various aspects of diffuse or nodular goiters are addressed in this book. The authors have been kind enough to include the best available information. The book is divided into sections for ease of reading.

N.K. Agrawal
Professor,
Department of Endocrinology and Metabolism,
Institute of Medical Sciences,
Banaras Hindu University,
Varanasi, India

Section 1

Overview

Chapter 1

Goiter: Overview of Aetiopathogenesis and Therapy

Dhananjaya Melkunte Shanthaiah, Piyush Gupta and Neeraj Kumar Agrawal

Abstract

The goiter was described in history for long time. Many luminaries suffered from it. The enlargement of thyroid is known as goiter, it can arise from various causes and each has separate aetiopathogenesis and treatment. As an overview for the book, this chapter delves into each aspect, whereas the details are in separate chapter.

Keywords: goiter, hypothyroidism, hyperthyroidism, thyroiditis, carcinoma thyroid

1. Introduction

Thyroid gland is a butterfly shaped organ lying in the anterior aspect of the neck. The major function of the gland is the production of thyroid hormones, namely Triiodothyronine and Tetraiodothyronine. These hormones are the major regulators of the various metabolic processes in the human body.

Various pathological processes affect the organ. One of the clinical manifestations of these pathological processes is enlargement of the gland. In general the abnormal enlargement of thyroid gland is defined as goiter by American thyroid association [1].

Historically goiter was mentioned in literature of various languages around the world. Ancient Indian physicians have described the condition called as Galaganda in detail in Ayurveda books written between fourteenth century BC and 400 A.D [2]. Many sculptures and paintings around the world have goiter being depicted suggest the prevalence of knowledge regarding goiter among the common people during those ages.

During 1600 BC Chinese used to treat the condition with the sea weed [3]. Even though ancient doctors use to treat the condition with sea weed, the exact pharmacological basis behind this treatment was understood only after the discovery of Iodine by Bernard Courtois in 1811 [4].

Association of iodine deficiency with goiter was first discovered during 19th century by various researchers like Lugol (1786–1851) and Coindet (1774–1834). But it was in the David Marine who proved requirement of iodine for normal thyroid function in a trial conducted between 1917 and 1922 in Ohio [5]. In 1835 Case of goiter with exophthalmos were described by Robert James Graves [6]. Thyroid hormone in pure form was extracted by Edward Kendall in 1914 at Mayo clinic [7].

Major progress occurred during twentieth century in management of Graves' disease with development of different treatment modalities like radioactive iodine and thionamides. Twenty-first century was marked with development of safer surgical practices and in depth understanding of the goiter pathology leading to better management of the condition.

2. Anatomy and embryology of thyroid gland

Thyroid gland is located anteriorly in lower neck and extending between C5 to T1 vertebrae. A normal adult thyroid gland is approximately 40–60 mm longitudinal and 13–18 mm AP diameter in size [8]. Mean ultrasound volume is around 7–10 ml and weighing of 9–21 g.

Microscopically the gland is divided into lobes and lobules. Lobules are further subdivided into follicles. These follicles are made up of principal (follicular) cells which are a type of epithelial cell. These cells produce colloid (iodo-thyroglobulin).

Other types of epithelial cells seen in gland are parafollicular cells (c cell) which lie adjacent to follicles. C cell produce calcitonin.

Thyroid gland development starts by third to fourth week of gestation and originates from primitive pharynx and the neural crest cells. The development begins as a diverticulum at the dorsum of tongue. This diverticulum forms hypoglossal duct which passes from foramen caecum to infrahyoid region. The supra hyoid part of thyroglossal duct degenerates whereas the infra hyoid part develops into thyroid gland.

The gland is supplied by superior thyroid artery, inferior thyroid artery and thyroidea ima. Venous drainage is provided by superior, middle and inferior thyroid vein.

The lymphatic drainage courses to prelaryngeal, pretracheal and paratracheal lymph node.

3. Classification of goiter

Goiter can be classified based on anatomically, etiologically, pathophysiologic ally and functionally (**Table 1** and **Figure 1**).

3.1 Dyshormonogenesis

Autosomal recessive disorders (exception DUOX 2 mutation). Enzymatic defect in one of the steps of thyroid hormone synthesis. The most common cause being the deficiency of thyroid peroxidase enzyme. Prevalence is more among females.

Anatomical classification of goiter
Cervical goiter
Retrosternal goiter
Intrathoracic goiter
Functional classification
Toxic goiter
Non-toxic goiter • Euthyroidism • Hypothyroidism
Morphological classification
Diffuse goiter
Nodular goiter • Solitary nodular goiter • Multinodular goiter

Table 1.
Anatomical, functional and morphological classification of goiter.

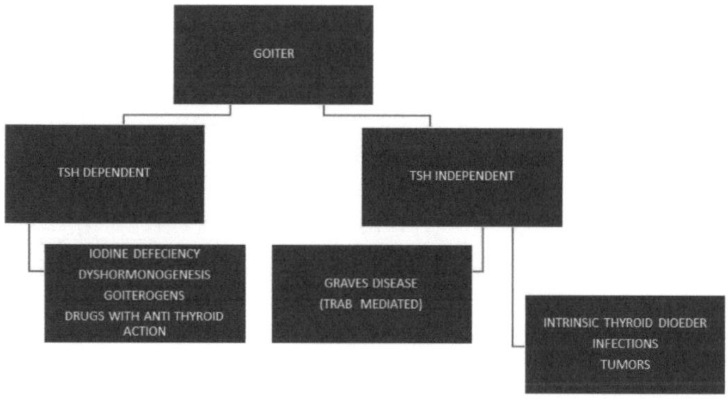

Figure 1.
Classification of goiter on the basis of pathophysiology.

Most of the cases present clinically before third decade with as earliest as in neonatal period with goiter and hypothyroidism. In Pendred syndrome dyshormonogenetic goiter is associated with deafness.

3.2 Dietary factors

3.2.1 Iodine deficiency

Twenty-nine percent of world population lives in area where soil is deficient in iodine, e.g., the Himalayan region in India. The most common cause of goiter worldwide is iodine deficiency. More than 30% of population having median urine iodine less than 20 mcg/l developed goiter [9]. Daily requirement of iodine is 100–150 mcg/day, but the requirement increases in pregnant and lactating women.

3.2.2 Dietary goitrogens

Soy and Millet contains flavonoids which impair thyroid peroxidase activity. Cyanogenic glucosides in Cassava, Lima beans compete for iodine uptake in thyroid follicles. Similarly cruciferous vegetables like cabbage cauliflower, broccoli contains glucosinolates which also competes with thyroidal iodine uptake.

3.3 Drugs causing goiter

Drugs like Lithium, Amiodarone apart from Antithyroid drugs are known to cause goiter. Rare causes include Interferon Alfa, Rifampicin, Phenytoin, and Phenobarbitone.

3.4 Hashimotos thyroiditis

The condition is named after Japanese physician Hakaru Hashimoto. This autoimmune thyroid disorder is characterized by diffuse lymphocytic infiltration of thyroid gland along with follicular destruction. Serologically the patients have high titer of anti-thyroglobulin and anti TPO antibodies. Hashimoto's thyroiditis is the next most common cause of hypothyroidism after iodine deficiency. But subset of patient may remain clinically and biochemically euthyroid for rest of the life. The condition has female to male prevalence ratio of 7:1.

3.5 Multinodular goiter

David Marine and Selwyn Taylor proposed that chronic intermittent stimulus leads to variable thyroid hyperplasia resulting in multinodular goiter [10]. Various factors including genetic heterogeneity of follicular cells, secondary elevation of TSH due to iodine deficiency, goitrogens, and inborn error of thyroid hormone synthesis are considered to be factors involved in pathogenesis of condition.

3.6 Infiltrative thyroid disorder

Various infiltrative disorders like amyloidosis, histiocytosis, cystinosis and sarcoidosis may affect thyroid gland.

3.7 Graves' disease

This autoimmune condition is characterized by presence of TRAB (TSH receptor autoantibodies) in the serum. The clinical feature ranges from hyperthyroidism, orbitopathy, dermopathy and goiter.

3.8 Thyroid adenoma

These are benign tumors, classified as either follicular (most common form) or papillary (rare) type. Adenomas may be hyper functioning when they are termed toxic adenoma. Follicular adenoma are histopathologically divided into Fetal (micro follicular), Colloid (macro follicular), Embryonal (atypical), Hurthle cell adenoma (oxyphil or oncocytic tumor) types. Among these with the exception of colloid type all other histopathological types have potential for micro invasion.

3.9 Thyroid malignancies

Thyroid malignancies are classified as papillary carcinoma (most common type), follicular carcinoma, medullary thyroid carcinoma, anaplastic carcinoma, thyroid lymphoma (rare) clinical features are explained below.

4. Pathophysiology of goiter

Thyroid stimulating hormone is the major trophic factor for thyroid gland. TSH acts on TSH receptors present on thyroid cells which are G protein coupled receptors. Downstream signaling leads to gene transcription leading to cell proliferation and differentiation (**Figure 2**).

The most common condition causing TSH dependent Goiter is iodine deficiency.

Goiter in chronic Hashimoto's thyroiditis is also secondary to elevated TSH levels.

In conditions like Graves' disease TSH receptors are stimulated by TSH stimulating antibodies Infection and neoplasia are examples for non-humoral causes of thyroid enlargement. Neoplastic enlargement occurs secondary to clonal expansion are usually are associated with underlying genetic alterations.

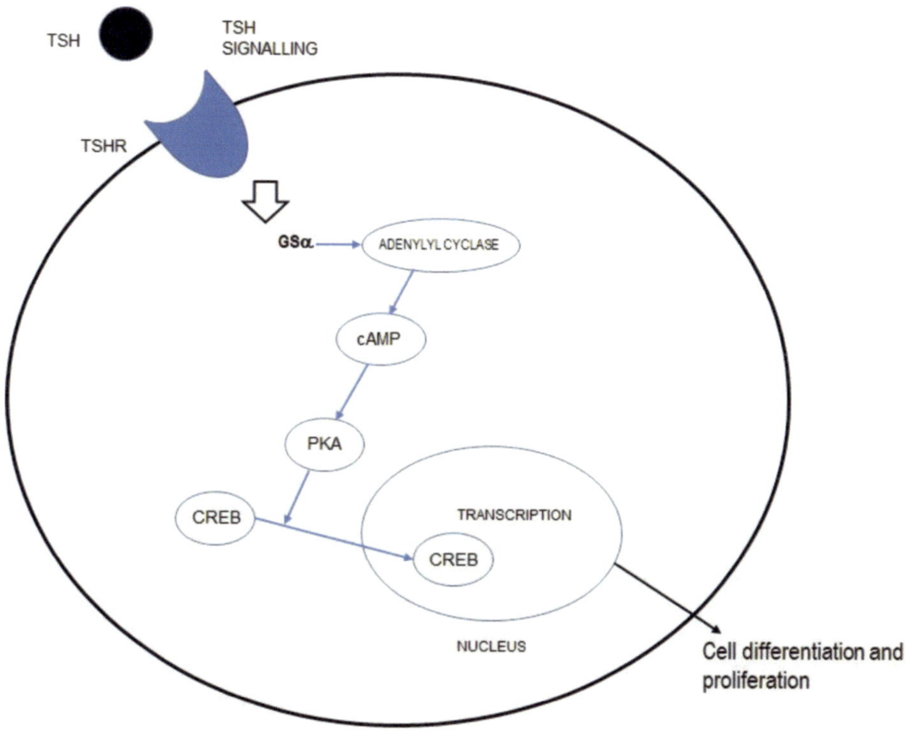

Figure 2.
TSH signaling pathway.

5. Differential diagnosis of swelling in anterior aspect of neck

5.1 Approach to patient with goiter

5.1.1 History and examination

Extensive history should be taken in all patients with goiter (**Table 2**).

Following points should be highlighted while taking history like place of residence (patients from high altitude areas iodine deficient), dietary iodine intake, family history of thyroid disorders, radiation exposure and any history of goitrogenic drugs intake.

1. Goiter
2. Neurogenic tumors
3. Thymoma
4. Bronchogenic cysts
5. Pericardial cysts
6. Lymphoma
7. Teratoma
8. Thyroglossal cyst

Table 2.
Differential diagnosis of swelling in anterior aspect of neck.

Major concern of nodular thyroid disorder is development of malignancy. Hence history regarding risk factors for malignancy like age (<20 and >60 years), male sex, previous radiation exposure, family history of thyroid malignancy, MEN 2A syndrome should be obtained.

5.2 Clinical evaluation

5.2.1 Physical examination

The thyroid examination is done with patient in sitting or standing position. Goiter is classified according to World Health Organization (WHO) classification [11] (**Table 3**).

Thyroid gland is palpated from behind the patient with neck relaxed and looked for size, consistency, nodules, and tenderness and lymphadenopathy.

Consistency of the enlarged gland helps in making diagnosis. Lesions which are hard for palpation suggest malignancy but rarely Reidel's thyroiditis may present like this. The gland feels rubbery in Hashimoto's thyroiditis. Diffuse tenderness can be elicited in sub-acute Thyroiditis.

Palpable thrill and hearing of bruit during auscultation over the gland suggest hypervacularity, it is seen in condition like Graves' disease.

During local examination one should look for lymphadenopathy and following group of lymph nodes should be examined (1) supraclavicular nodes, (2) anterior cervical chain lymph nodes, (3) posterior cervical chain lymph nodes, and (4) submental lymph nodes.

5.2.1.1 Pemberton's maneuver

The patient is advised to rise both the arm till they touch the face on respective sides. The test is considered positive if patient develops facial plethora. Thyroid gland obstructing thoracic inlet which lead to venous obstruction is considered to be the underlying mechanism.

Grade 0: No goiter is palpable or visible.
Grade 1: Palpable goiter, not visible when neck is held in normal position
Grade 2: A clearly swollen neck (also visible in normal position of the neck) that is consistent with a goiter on palpation

Table 3.
WHO classification of goiter.

Increased sweating	**Onycholysis**
Hyperpigmentation	Thinning of the hair
Systolic hypertension	Increase appetite
Weight loss	Palpitation
Heat intolerance	Insomnia
Hyper defecation	Menstrual irregularity oligo-/hypomenorrhea
Eye: lid retraction, lid lag, exophthalmos, ophthalmoplegia	

Table 4.
Symptoms and signs of hyperthyroidism.

General	Dermatological	Neuromuscular
• Lethargy	• Dry flaky skin and hair	• Aches and pains
• Somnolence	• Myxedema	• Muscle stiffness
• Weight gain	• Malar flushes	• Carpel tunnel syndrome
• Cold Intolerance	• Vitiligo	• Hoarseness
Cardiovascular	• Carotenemia	• Cerebellar ataxia
• Bradycardia	Gastro-intestinal	• Delayed deep tendon reflex
• Angina	• Constipation	• Myotonia
• Congestive heart failure	• Ileus	• Depression
• Pericardial Effusion	• Ascites	• Psychosis
Hematological	Reproductive system	
• Anemia	• Infertility	
	• Menorrhagia	

Table 5.
Signs and symptoms of hypothyroidism.

General examination includes looking signs of hyperthyroidism, hypothyroidism and metastatic involvement of different organs in suspected thyroid malignancy.

Signs and symptoms of hyperthyroidism and hypothyroidism are enlisted in **Tables 4** and 5 respectively.

Symptoms of thyroid malignancy: Most commonly manifest as solitary nodule which are usually painless in nature. Malignant conversion of thyroid nodules is more common among males than females. Hoarseness of voice and dysphagia suggest local involvement of recurrent laryngeal nerve and digestive tract.

Malignant nodules on palpation range from soft to hard consistency. Regional lymphadenopathy suggests lymph node metastasis.

5.2.2 Investigation

5.2.2.1 Thyroid function test

Thyroid function test is evaluated starting with measurement of measurement of serum TSH level. If TSH level are less than normal values then next step is to measure T3 and. Normal T3 and T4 level (total T4: 4.5–12.5 μg/dL, free T4: 0.8–1.7 ng/dL, total T3:0.8–2.0 ng/ml, free T3: 2.3–4.2 pg./mL) suggest subclinical hyperthyroidism whereas elevated T3 and T4 level suggest overt hyperthyroidism. Both overt and subclinical hyperthyroidism suggest Graves' disease or toxic MNG.

If TSH levels are less than normal value then next step is to measure T4 level. Subclinical hypothyroidism is considered when value of TSH levels between 5 and 10 μU/ml with normal T4 level. Iodine deficiency and Hashimoto's thyroiditis are the most common cause of subclinical or overt hypothyroidism.

5.2.2.2 Thyroid peroxidase antibodies

Presence of the antibody in serum suggest autoimmune thyroid disorder

5.2.2.3 Thyroid ultrasound

Even though all patients with enlarged thyroid gland requires sonographic assessment to rule out malignancy, risk decreases in patients having TSH below normal or in low normal range. There are certain indications which make ultrasound assessment mandatory like palpable solitary nodule, palpable multinodular goiter, and suspicion of nodule in patient with difficult neck palpation, rapid growth of a goiter, thyroid asymmetry, firm consistency, tenderness, normal TSH and negative TPO antibodies.

5.2.2.4 Fine-needle aspiration cytology

Indications for FNAC include rapid growth of the swelling which suggest malignant transformation, signs of inflammation (abscess formation) and nodules with indeterminate or suspicious features (ultrasound proven).

5.2.2.5 Computed tomography of neck

Computed tomography of neck not usually advised is required rarely to assess the extension of large cervical goiters and sub sternal goiters.

5.2.2.6 Technetium-99 m (^{99m}Tc) thyroid scans/radioiodine uptake scans

Routine use of thyroid scintigraphy is not indicated in the assessment of goiter. A hot area in scintigraphy suggest benign lesion which can be of help to rule out malignant lesions when FNAC report of the thyroid nodules are equivocal. When TSH level is low and clinical features are suggestive of hyperthyroidism technetium-99 scan/Radio iodine uptake scan are useful to differentiate between Graves' disease, thyroiditis and toxic adenoma.

6. Treatment

Treatment of goiter depends on whether TSH levels are normal or abnormal.

If TSH is elevated than normal, Levothyroxine supplementation is given for patient with overt hypothyroidism starting with a dose of 1.6 mcg/kg body weight per day in non-pregnant adults.

There are certain Indications for treatment of subclinical hypothyroidism like Anti-TPO positivity, menstrual irregularity, infertility, chronic kidney disease, pregnancy.

If TSH is less than normal range then the treatment modality depends on the nature of the illness in Graves' disease we have got three effective treatment modalities, i.e., thionamides (anti-thyroid drugs), radioiodine or surgery. Starting dose of Methimazole ranges from 10 to 40 mg per day in divided doses initially followed by single daily dose-Beta blockers are used for relief of tachycardia in non-asthmatic patients.

In multinodular goiter and toxic adenoma treatment modality is either radioiodine ablation surgery.

Iodine radioisotope I-131 is usually used for radioiodine ablation. It takes 6–18 weeks for thyroid tissue ablation post radioiodine administration. Treatment of subclinical hyperthyroidism is considered in patient older than age of 65 years and patient with other comorbidities like heart disease, osteoporosis, and post-menopausal women not on HRT.

Surgery is indicated in patients with large goiters with compressive symptoms, malignancy, and failed medical therapy.

7. Conclusions

The goiter is a known disorder affecting females more than males. It has various etiologies classified depending on the levels of TSH. The treatment of goiter is according to the etiology.

Conflict of interest

The authors declare no conflict of interest.

Author details

Dhananjaya Melkunte Shanthaiah[1], Piyush Gupta[2] and Neeraj Kumar Agrawal[1*]

1 Department of Endocrinology and Metabolism, Institute of Medical Sciences - BHU, India

2 Department of General Surgery, University of Massachusetts, Worcester, USA

*Address all correspondence to: drnkavns@gmail.com

References

[1] Definition of Goiter. Available from: https://www.thyroid.org/goiter [Accessed: 04 June 2019]

[2] Leoutsakos V. A short history of the thyroid gland. Hormones. 2004;**3**:268-271

[3] Sarkar S, Banerjee S, Sarkar R, Sikder B. A review on the history of 'Thyroid Surgery'. The Indian Journal of Surgery. 2016;**78**(1):32-36. DOI: 10.1007/s12262-015-1317-5

[4] Zimmermann MB. Research on iodine deficiency and goiter in the 19th and early 20th centuries. The Journal of Nutrition. 2008;**138**(11):2060-2063

[5] Carpenter KJ. David Marine and the problem of goiter. The Journal of Nutrition. 2005;**135**(4):675-680

[6] Ellis H. Robert Graves: Graves' disease of the thyroid. Journal of Perioperative Practice. 2012;**22**(5):176-176. DOI: 10.1177/175045891202200507

[7] Lindholm J, Laurberg P. Hypothyroidism and thyroid substitution: Historical aspects. Journal of Thyroid Research. 2011;**2011**:809341. DOI: 10.4061/2011/809341

[8] Chaudhary V, Bano S. Thyroid ultrasound. Indian Journal of Endocrinology and Metabolism. 2013;**17**(2):219-227. DOI: 10.4103/2230-8210.109667

[9] WHO, UNICEF, ICCIDD. Assessment of Iodine Deficiency Disorders and Monitoring Their Elimination. Geneva: WHO; 2001

[10] Medeiros-Neto G. Multinodular goiter [Updated: September 26, 2016]. In: Feingold KR, Anawalt B, Boyce A, et al., editors. Endotext [Internet]. South Dartmouth, MA: MDText.com, Inc.; 2000

[11] Azizi F et al. Assessment, Monitoring and Evaluation of Iodine Deficiency Disorders in the Middle East and Eastern Mediterranean Region. Teheran: Sara Publications; 2002

Section 2

Goitrous Hypothyroidism

Chapter 2

Autoimmune Basis of Sub Clinical Hypothyroidism in Pregnancy

Prakruti Dash and Rajlaxmi Tiwari

Abstract

Effects of overt hypothyroidism on pregnancy outcomes and fetal development are well established and treatment protocol is reputable. Subclinical hypothyroidism poses a major health problem in pregnancy. Requirement of iodine increases in pregnancy as demand for synthesis of excess thyroid hormones is there during pregnancy. This is because of fetal dependency on maternal thyroid hormones till 12 weeks of gestation as fetal thyroid tissue is not matured enough to produce adequate hormones for the growing fetus. Hence, dietary iodine deficiency or intake of excess goitrogens in diet can be the major cause of overt and subclinical hypothyroidism in pregnancy. Apart from this autoimmune basis of overt and sub clinical hypothyroidism is also equally important in pregnant women. Data accumulating shows presence of antibodies like anti TPO antibody (anti thyroperoxidase antibody) and anti Tg antibody (anti thyroglobulin antibody) in pregnancy which is associated with increased prevalence of overt and sub clinical hypothyroidism and aggravation of the symptoms associated with it. Studies also document that pregnancy related complications are more prevalent in presence of these autoimmune antibodies. Hence, management of subclinical hypothyroidism in pregnancy also differs in positive and negative cases of anti TPO antibody and anti-Tg antibody.

Keywords: sub-clinical hypothyroidism, pregnancy, obstetric outcome, autoimmunity, anti thyroperoxidase antibody (anti TPO antibody), anti-thyroglobulin antibody (anti Tg antibody), assisted fertilization

1. Introduction

Subclinical hypothyroidism (SCH), frequently observed in pregnancy is defined as high TSH with normal T4 and T3 level. The growing fetus is entirely dependent on mother thyroid hormones in the first 12 weeks; hence, any abnormalities during this period should be detected early and preventive measures initiated as decreased thyroid hormones is known to affect the mother and the fetus adversely.

Presence of anti-TPO antibody is a major risk factor for progression to overt hypothyroidism. After widespread use of fortified Iodine rich food and extra supplementation of iodine in pregnancy, the knowledge and prevalence of autoimmune clinical and subclinical hypothyroidism with presence of various antibodies against thyroid tissues and metabolic factors gains more importance. Adverse obstetric and fetal outcomes particularly attributed to anti TPO antibodies makes its study even more clinically relevant. It is important to know the burden of anti-TPO antibody associated SCH cases due to their differences in management.

Parameter	Changes during pregnancy	Normal values (up to)
TSH	Reaches nadir during first trimester; then plateaus	4.0 mIU/L
T4	Increases in first trimester; then plateaus	150 ng/mL
fT4	Unchanged	30 pg/mL
T3	Increases in first trimester; then plateaus	2 ng/mL
fT3	Unchanged	4 pg/mL

Table 1.
Normal levels of thyroid hormones and TSH in pregnancy [1].

1.1 Anatomical, physiological and biochemical adaption of thyroid gland to pregnancy

A palpable increase in size of the thyroid gland is observed in normal pregnancy which is also associated with a bruit [1]. There is an established increased renal clearance of iodide leading to increased thyroid iodide clearance with associated raised uptake of ^{131}Iodide by the thyroid glands during pregnancy. This results in a relative iodine deficient status in the pregnant mother. There is also an increase in TBG (thyroid hormone binding globulin) for which total thyroxine exhibits a raised value but free thyroxine and free triiodothyronine (fT3) is mostly normal (**Table 1**).

1.2 Regulation of synthesis of thyroid hormones in pregnancy

The synthesis of thyroid hormones is regulated by HPT axis, i.e., hypothalamus-pituitary-thyroid axis. The TRH released from hypothalamus acts positively on pituitary gland which releases TSH [1]. The TSH in turn stimulates the thyroid gland to synthesize and release T4 and T3. The thyroid gland gives negative feedback signal to hypothalamus and pituitary and thus excess of its synthesis is controlled and regulated. During pregnancy, in addition to the normal regulatory mechanisms, hCG also plays a significant role in regulation of thyroid hormone synthesis. hCG mostly the asialo-hCG fraction secreted from the placenta is known to have weak TSH simulating action and this plays an important role in maintaining the thyroid hormone levels, whose demand is increased in pregnancy due to fetal dependency on mother's thyroid hormones almost exclusively up to 12 weeks of gestation and hCG acts by contributing to thyrotropic action of placenta. This also results in mild hyperthyroidism status in early pregnancy.

2. Anti-thyroid antibodies to thyroid antigens

2.1 Anti TPO antibody

Polyclonal antibodies directed against some epitopes of thyroperoxidase molecule are present in the blood of some healthy individuals and patients having auto immune thyroid disorders [1–3]. Anti-TPO antibodies from auto immune thyroid patients act as competitive inhibitors of enzymatic activity though those from healthy subjects are not seen to block thyroperoxidase [4, 5]. These antibodies mostly belong to IgG class, more often IgG1and IgG4 subtypes [6]. Prevalence of anti-TPO antibodies are more common than other anti-thyroid antibodies and more symbolic for thyroid hormone imbalance. Excess of oxidative stress markers in blood are seen with anti-TPO antibodies indicating it to be an inducer of oxidative stress [7]. Apart from hypothyroid patients, anti-TPO antibodies are also detected in Graves' disease patients. These antibodies possess the potential of crossing the placenta barrier to variable extent [8], though its effect on the neonate is debatable.

Few studies document that children born to anti TPO antibody positive pregnant women supposedly suffer from compromised motor and neuropsychological development [9]. There can be behavioral problems, attention deficit disorders in the off springs associated with raised titers of anti TPO antibody in the mothers during pregnancy [10]. Couple of literatures substantiate that children of anti TPO antibody positive mothers have lower brain to body mass ratio, decreased weight of brain and smaller head circumference compared to those of anti TPO antibody negative mothers [11, 12].

As the influence and outcome on off springs of increased anti TPO antibody concentration during pregnancy is of greater significance, longer follow up studies is required to gather more data on this important clinical aspect of neuropsychological development of the children.

2.2 Anti-thyroglobulin antibody

Polyclonal anti thyroglobulin (Tg) antibodies are found in the serum of healthy subjects whereas oligoclonal antibodies are seen in patients having auto immune thyroid disorders. It has been hypothesized that normal blood levels of Tg induce self-tolerance in T cells as low levels of antigens are usually responsible for development of self-tolerance. But this self-tolerance is not seen in case of B cell activity resulting in healthy individuals having very low levels of anti-Tg antibodies which is usually below detection limits. Higher levels of Tg following tissue damage, or due to conformation alteration of the Tg molecule in presence of high iodine levels, or in presence of very high TSH levels, there is alteration in the titers of the anti-Tg antibody. The anti-Tg antibodies are predominantly of IgG4 though minor proportions of IgA and IgM class are also seen. The functional consequence of anti-Tg antibodies is hitherto not known. Circulating antibodies were detected in healthy young subjects and in people >60 years of age to an extent of 10–15%. Presence of anti-Tg antibodies have been documented in auto immune thyroid disorders, Graves' disease and in patients with non-thyroid immune disorders. These antibodies like anti TPO antibodies can cross the placenta barrier but its effects are not very substantially known [1].

2.3 Thyroid hormone receptor antibodies

These antibodies bind to thyroid cell membrane at/near TSH receptor and mimics the action of TSH as "occupied" receptor. This leads to excess thyroxin synthesis by the gland which escapes feedback control mechanisms. It is demonstrated frequently in Grave's disease-also known as long acting thyroid stimulator (LATS) antibodies.

Excess of synthesis of thyroid hormones is known as hyperthyroidism and deficiency leads to hypothyroidism. Both the conditions are associated with deleterious effects to various metabolic processes of the body [1].

3. Thyroid hormones and pregnancy

Thyroid hormones T4 and T3 affect almost every metabolic processes of the body. Pregnancy is considered to be a physiologically altered state of metabolism as the body tries to cater to the needs of the growing fetus. There is an increased need of thyroid hormones in pregnancy as the developing fetus is completely dependent on maternal thyroid hormones till 12 weeks of gestation. Hence, the gland becomes over stimulated and hyperactive to secrete more T4 and T3 to meet the increased demand and this is brought about through hypothalamus-pituitary-thyroid axis regulatory mechanisms. Thyroxin and TBG (thyroid binding globulins) levels rise in pregnancy along with a simultaneous decrease in TSH (thyroid stimulating hormone) level [13]. A placental deiodinase enzyme also results in more thyroid hormone synthesis in pregnancy [14–16]. hCG is known to have a TSH simulating effect and hence attributes to raise the thyroid hormone synthesis to meet the increased demand via its thyrotrophic effect [17]. Absolute fetal dependency on mother's thyroid hormones can result in adverse obstetric and fetal outcome if the increased demand for T4 and T3 is not met adequately in the first 12 weeks of gestation [18]. There has also been documented evidences that proper placental development is also dependent on thyroid hormones and lack of it can result in improper placenta formation [19] with adverse obstetric outcomes like abruptio placentae, preeclampsia, miscarriages, preterm delivery, low birth weight (LBW), IUGR (intrauterine growth retardation) and small for gestational age babies (SGA) [20–22]. Impaired intellectual development of off springs of hyper/hypothyroid mothers has also been documented [23].

3.1 Thyroid hormones and its effects on obstetric outcome

Various studies have registered in their findings that placenta has strong affinity for T3 and is dependent on thyroid hormones for its growth. Triiodothyronine/ T3 is plays a significant role in placental trophoblastic growth by its likely effect on growth factors like EGF (epidermal growth factor) and hormone like 17 beta estradiol [19, 24, 25]. Small for gestational age babies (SGA) and intra uterine growth retardation of fetus (IUGR) are most likely results of impaired growth of placental trophoblasts [26, 27]. Fetal thyroid hormones have been found to be decreased in IUGR babies compared to gestation matched normal fetal serum. Inflammation associated with impaired uteroplacental circulation are registered to be causative factors for development of serious disorders like eclampsia and preeclampsia in pregnancy. These situations are also documented to be associated with increased oxidative stress by various studies [28]. Hence various studies now put inflammation under major focus in development of preeclampsia and pre-term labor in pregnancy. Thyroid hormones act on DNA and regulate expression of various genes which also includes genes associated with inflammation. As inflammation is now considered to be an important causative factor for development of pre-eclampsia, thyroid hormones are also corroborated by various studies to be responsible for this [29]. Analysis of maternal and cord blood has validated this hypothesis and revealed a low T4 with raised TSH level in preeclampsia cases which has also been linked with placental inadequacy.

Various studies have also found an association of gestational diabetes mellitus (GDM) with impaired thyroid status. Inverse correlation between metformin and TSH value further strengthens this association. Thus, screening of all pregnant women for thyroid function along with anti TPO antibody measurement has been advised by many studies, particularly in "at risk "cases of GDM [30–33]. Both thyroid dysfunction and diabetes mellitus are known to adversely affect obstetric and fetal outcome and now gradually gathering data proves that very often both the conditions coexist in pregnancy depicting an association between them and hence early screening, intervention and timely management is advocated by various studies [34–37].

3.2 Pregnancy and clinical/subclinical hypothyroidism

The need for iodine increases in pregnancy (daily requirement of iodine –150–200 μg/day, 250 μg/day in pregnancy) leading to an iodine deficient status if not adequately supplemented. Apart from iodine deficiency, the other most common factor for thyroid hormone deficiency has been attributed to anti-TPO antibodies. Hypothyroidism is registered to be more prevalent in Asian countries compared to their Western counterparts. As such thyroid disorders have wide geographical variations attributed to dietary factors, level of various goitrogens in diet and their consumption level, deficiencies of micronutrients like selenium, iron and most importantly iodine. Autoimmune thyroid diseases are also more prevalent in Asian countries and accumulating literatures suggest it to be more substantial in Indian population with greater prevalence of anti TPO antibody positivity.

High TSH level with normal T4 level is known as subclinical hypothyroidism (SCH). Subclinical hypothyroidism is one of the most common type of thyroid dysfunction that is found to be associated with pregnancy [38, 39]. The increased need of thyroid hormones to meet the extra demand by the growing fetus in the first 12 weeks of gestation is dealt by hCG due to its thyrotrophic action as discussed earlier and also via hypothalamus-pituitary-thyroid axis regulation which usually results in small painless enlargement, i.e., goiter formation in pregnant women [1]. This also results in increased need of iodine in pregnancy.

Hence, endemic areas of iodine deficiency have shown a higher prevalence of clinical or subclinical hypothyroidism in general and in particular in pregnant women. Because of increased thyroid hormone production, increased renal iodine excretion, and fetal iodine requirements, dietary iodine requirements are higher in pregnancy than they are for non-pregnant adults. The requirement of iodine is 250 μg/day in pregnancy. Recommendation by American Thyroid Association (ATA) is women who are planning pregnancy or currently pregnant, should supplement their diet with a daily oral supplement that contains 150 μg of iodine in the form of potassium iodide [40]. This should optimally start 3 months in advance of planned pregnancy.

3.3 Hypothyroidism and autoimmunity in pregnancy

However, apart from iodine deficiency, the other most significant cause of hypothyroidism in recent times is presence of anti thyroperoxidase antibody, i.e., anti TPO antibody and anti Tg (anti thyroglobulin) antibody in the serum. The thyroperoxidase enzyme as described above is highly essential for oxidation of trapped iodine and its incorporation into tyrosine molecule for synthesis of thyroxin. Anti TPO antibody destroys the thyroperoxidase enzyme and hence prevents the iodination of tyrosine molecule and overall synthesis of thyroxin is hampered resulting in hypothyroidism. This autoimmune basis of hypothyroidism is now more relevant after iodine deficiency has been tackled by fortification of food products with iodine/with iodine supplementation as potassium iodide. In pregnancy, immune regulatory cytokines and cells are present in the mother's circulatory system and accumulate in the decidua and can modify autoimmune responses influencing the symptoms of autoimmune disease [41].

Presence of anti-TPO antibody is a major risk factor for progression to overt hypothyroidism. Various studies reveal a prevalence of 2–17% of euthyroid pregnant women being anti-TPO antibody positive. Still data from Indian scenario is extremely limited. TPO antibodies are able to cross the placenta. At the time of delivery, cord blood anti TPO Ab levels strongly correlate with third-trimester maternal anti TPO antibody concentrations [8]. However, concrete documentation of maternal passage of either anti TPO antibodies or anti Tg antibodies affecting the fetal thyroid function is still debatable [9–12].

It has been documented that euthyroid pregnant women who are positive for thyroid peroxidase autoantibody (anti TPO antibody) also are at increased risk of various complications of pregnancy including miscarriage, preterm birth, pregnancy-induced hypertension (PIH), intrauterine death (IUD), and intrauterine growth retardation (IUGR) [42, 43].

A number of etiologies have been hypothesized as the cause of the relationship between various pregnancy related complications like miscarriage, IUGR, pre-eclampsia, pre term delivery and autoimmune thyroid antibodies. To enumerate a few: (a) prior presence of a restrained degree of hypothyroidism, (b) thyroid antibodies reflecting an immunological imbalance inclining towards auto immunity in the pregnant female, (c) direct effects of thyroid autoantibodies on the placenta or the fertilized ovum. The above hypotheses have been corroborated by the observation of higher levels of TSH within the normal range noted in various meta-analysis studies indicating a milder degree of thyroid failure in euthyroid pregnant women with thyroid auto antibodies positivity [41, 44–46].

3.4 Autoimmune hypothyroidism and development of goiter in pregnancy

Pregnancy is considered to be a goitrogenic status, particularly in the Iodine deficiency scenario. Increased need of thyroid hormones, TSH simulating actions of beta HCG with super added iodine deficiency actually leads to volumetric increase in the gland and not just vascular engorgement which also has been biochemically corroborated by observations of high serum Thyroglobulin levels, more T3 secretion and small rise in basal TSH level at delivery. Studies supports that there is actual goiter formation in pregnancy which can be tackled to a measurable extent by adequate iodine supplementation [47].

Presence of anti TPO antibodies is mostly associated with Hashimoto's thyroiditis, Graves' disease, nodular goiter and thyroid carcinoma [1]. Anti TPO antibody positivity in pregnancy is mostly associated with overt or subclinical hypothyroidism during pregnancy sometimes associated with a goiter which is often painless. Post-delivery, there are incidences of postpartum thyroiditis with a milder form of Graves' disease lacking the typical symptomatic features which after a few months, changes to hypothyroidism and development of small painless goiter [1, 48, 49].

4. Reference limits for diagnosis of hypothyroidism in pregnancy

It is important to know the burden of anti-TPO antibody associated SCH cases due to their differences in management. This is even more important in case of pregnant women as presence of anti TPO antibody makes them more vulnerable to clinical hypothyroidism and hence its detection at early pregnancy helps in its better management. The management for pregnant women with subclinical hypothyroidism with anti TPO Ab positive and negative differs from each other.

Setting the reference limits for thyroid hormones and TSH in pregnancy is a debatable fact due to different laboratories giving different values and there is gross geographical variation too. Guidelines of the American Thyroid Association for the Diagnosis and Management of Thyroid Disease during Pregnancy and Postpartum (ATA 2011) recommends a trimester specific range of TSH in pregnancy which is lower than in normal adult, i.e., first trimester: 0.1–2.5 mIU/L, second trimester: 0.2–3.0 mIU/L, third trimester: 0.3–3.0 mIU/L [40]. However, the recent guidelines

	TSH value	T4/T3	Anti TPO	Therapy with LT4
1	Within the pregnancy-specific reference range or <4.0 mIU/L (if specific reference range unavailable)	Normal	Negative	Not recommended
2	TSH >10.0 mU/L	Normal	Negative	Strong recommendation
3	TSH >2.5 mU/L and below the upper limit of the pregnancy-specific reference range	Normal	Positive	Weak recommendation
4	TSH greater than the upper limit of the pregnancy-specific reference range but below 10.0 mU/L	Normal	Negative	Weak recommendation
5	TSH greater than pregnancy-specific reference range or >4.0 mIU/L (if specific reference range unavailable)	Normal	Positive	Strong recommendation

Table 2.
Recommendations by ATA 2017 guidelines regarding management of sub clinical hypothyroidism in pregnancy [50].

of ATA recommend "When available, population- and trimester-specific reference ranges for serum TSH during pregnancy should be defined by a provider's institute or laboratory and should represent the typical population for whom care is provided. Reference ranges should be defined in healthy anti TPO Ab-negative pregnant women with optimal iodine intake and without thyroid illness. If internal or transferable pregnancy-specific TSH reference ranges are not available, an upper reference limit of ~4.0 mIU/L may be used" (ATA-2017) [50]. In the absence of accredited trimester specific reference ranges for thyroid hormones and TSH levels in pregnancy in India, the current practice is to use the reference limits set by ATA as per 2017 guidelines [50].

4.1 Management of overt and subclinical hypothyroidism in pregnancy

Recent guidelines of ATA recommends regular monitoring of thyroid status in women with overt and subclinical hypothyroidism (treated or untreated) or those at risk for hypothyroidism (e.g., patients who are euthyroid but anti TPO antibody or anti Tg antibody positive, post-hemithyroidectomy, or treated with radioactive iodine) with a serum TSH measurement approximately every 4 weeks until completion of second trimester and at least once near 30 weeks gestation [50]. Sub clinical hypothyroidism in anti TPO antibody negative and positive cases in pregnancy are differently managed with levothyroxine (LT4) as per the recommendations of ATA 2017 guidelines [50] (**Table 2**).

5. Thyroid auto antibodies and assisted fertilization

Recently, some researchers speculated that assisted conception in women positive for anti-thyroid antibodies had poor outcome of *in vitro* fertilization, even if they were euthyroid. Studies do document that anti thyroid antibodies positive patients had low fertilization rate, implantation rate, and pregnancy rate and high abortion rate. Regarding the question how these antibodies interfered with fertilization, embryo development as well as implantation potential still remains unanswered. The hypothesis is that the antibodies may bind to either the surface of the egg and/or embryo and interfere with fertilization and subsequent embryo development. Alternatively, the presence of the auto antibodies in the endometrial tissue may exert detrimental effect on embryo implantation leading to early pregnancy loss [51–54].

6. Conclusion

More and more evidences worldwide have pointed towards anti TPO antibody to be associated with clinical and subclinical hypothyroidism with adverse obstetric and fetal outcomes. As the management differs for subclinical hypothyroidism in anti TPO antibody positive and negative pregnant women hence more studies should be undertaken pertinent to different geographical areas regarding the prevalence of autoantibodies and their effect on pregnancy and on the off springs in the long term. The trimester specific reference ranges for different areas should also be specified with larger cohort of studies particularly for countries like India where there are wide geographical and ethnic variations. The area where there is severe lacking of data with respect to India is regarding the effects of autoimmune subclinical hypothyroidism on the obstetric, fetal outcomes and most importantly on the off springs in the long run. Hence, longer follow-up studies with larger cohorts is necessary to gather more evidences regarding this important endocrinal disorder in pregnancy in India.

Author details

Prakruti Dash* and Rajlaxmi Tiwari
Department of Biochemistry, All India Institute of Medical Sciences, Bhubaneswar, Odisha, India

*Address all correspondence to: dashdrprakruti@gmail.com

References

[1] Cooper DS, Ladenson PW. The Thyroid Gland. Greenspan's Basic and Clinical Endocrinology. 9th ed. China: The McGraw-Hill Companies; 2011. pp. 163-226

[2] Volpe R. Immunology of human thyroid disease. In: Volpe R, editor. Autoimmune Diseases of the Endocrine System. Boca Raton, FL: CRC Press; 1990. pp. 73-240

[3] Stathatos N, Daniels GH. Autoimmune thyroid disease. Current Opinion in Rheumatology. 2014;**24**:70-75

[4] Kohno Y, Yamaguchi F, Saito K, Niimi H, Nishikawa T, Hosoya T. Anti-thyroid peroxidase antibodies in sera from healthy subjects and from patients with chronic thyroiditis: Differences in the ability to inhibit thyroid peroxidase activities. Clinical and Experimental Immunology. 1991;**85**:459-463. DOI: 10.1111/j.1365-2249.1991.tb05749.x

[5] Kaczur V, Vereb G, Molnar I, Krajczar G, Kiss E, Farid NR, et al. Effect of anti-thyroid peroxidase (TPO) antibodies on TPO activity measured by chemiluminescence assay. Clinical Chemistry. 1997;**43**:1392-1396

[6] Xie LD, Gao Y, Li MR, Lu GZ, Guo XH. Distribution of immunoglobulin G subclasses of anti-thyroid peroxidase antibody in sera from patients with Hashimoto's thyroiditis with different thyroid functional status. Clinical and Experimental Immunology. 2008;**154**:172-176. DOI: 10.1111/j.1365-2249.2008.03756.x

[7] Ruggeri RM, Vicchio TM, Cristani M, Certo R, Caccamo D, Alibrandi A, et al. Oxidative stress and advanced glycation end products in Hashimoto's thyroiditis. Thyroid. 2016;**26**:504-511. DOI: 10.1089/thy.2015.059228

[8] Seror J, Amand G, Guibourdenche J, Ceccaldi P-F, Luton D. Anti-TPO antibodies diffusion through the placental barrier during pregnancy. PLoS ONE. 2014;**9**(1):e84647. DOI: 10.1371/journal.pone.0084647

[9] Li Y, Shan Z, Teng W, et al. Abnormalities of maternal thyroid function during pregnancy affect neuropsychological development of their children at 25-30 months. Clinical Endocrinology. 2010;**72**(6):825-829

[10] Ghassabian A, Bongers-Schokking JJ, De Rijke YB, et al. Maternal thyroid autoimmunity during pregnancy and the risk of attention deficit/hyperactivity problems in children: The Generation R study. Thyroid. 2012;**22**(2):178-186

[11] Roneé EW, Hamisu MS, Maureen WG, Dagne G, O'Rourke K, Alfred KM. Impact of maternal thyroperoxidase status on fetal body and brain size. Thyroid. 2003;**3**:340-356

[12] Lafranchi SH, Haddow JE, Hollowell JG. Is thyroid inadequacy during gestation a risk factor for adverse pregnancy and developmental outcomes? Thyroid. 2005;**15**:60-71

[13] Lin KH, Lee HY, Shih CH, Yen CC, Chen SL, Yang RC, et al. Plasma protein regulation by thyroid hormone. The Journal of Endocrinology. 2003;**179**:367-377

[14] Glinoer D, DeNayer P, Bourdoux P, Lemone M, Robyn C, Van Steirteghem A, et al. Regulation of maternal thyroid during pregnancy. The Journal of Clinical Endocrinology and Metabolism. 1990;**71**:276-287. DOI: 10.1210/jcem-71-2-276

[15] Guillaume J, Schussler GC, Goldman J, Wassel P, Bach L. Components of the total serum thyroid

hormone concentrations during pregnancy: High free thyroxine and blunted thyrotropin (TSH) response to TSH-releasing hormone in the first trimester. The Journal of Clinical Endocrinology and Metabolism. 1985;**60**:678-684. DOI: 10.1210/jcem-60-4-678

[16] Kwakkel J, Surovtseva OV, de Vries EM, Stap J, Fliers E, Boelen A. A novel role for the thyroid hormone-activating enzyme type 2 deiodinase in the inflammatory response of macrophages in pregnancy. Placenta. 2013;**34**:395-400. DOI: 10.1016/j.placenta.2013.02.009

[17] Yoshimura M, Hershman JM. Thyrotropic action of human chorionic gonadotropin. Thyroid. 1995;**5**:425-434. DOI: 10.1089/thy.1995.5.425

[18] Utiger RD. Maternal hypothyroidism and fetal development. The New England Journal of Medicine. 1999;**341**:601-602. DOI: 10.1056/NEJM199908193410809

[19] Banovac K, Ryan EA, O'Sullivan MJ. Triiodothyronine nuclear binding sites in human placenta and decidua. Placenta. 1986;**7**:543-549. DOI: 10.1016/S0143-4004(86)80140-0

[20] Fisher DA. Thyroid function in very low birth weight infants. Clinical Endocrinology. 1997;**47**:419-421. DOI: 10.1046/j.1365-2265.1997.3021106.x

[21] Davis LE, Leveno KJ, Cunningham FG. Hypothyroidism complicating pregnancy. Obstetrics and Gynecology. 1988;**72**(1):108-112

[22] Leung AS, Millar LK, Koonings PP, Montoro M, Mestman JH. Perinatal outcome in hypothyroid pregnancies. Obstetrics and Gynecology. 1993;**81**(3):349-353. DOI: 10.1016/0020-7292(93)90343-u

[23] Haddow JE, Palomaki GE, Allan WC, Williams JR, Knight GJ, Gagnon J, et al. Maternal thyroid deficiency during pregnancy and subsequent neuropsychological development of the child. The New England Journal of Medicine. 1999;**341**:549-555. DOI: 10.1056/NEJM199908193410801

[24] Oki N, Matsuo H, Nakago S, Murakoshi H, Laoag-Fernandez JB, Maruo T. Effects of 3, 5, 3′-triiodothyronine on the invasive potential and the expression of integrins and matrix metalloproteinases in cultured early placental extravillous trophoblasts. The Journal of Clinical Endocrinology and Metabolism. 2004;**89**:5213-5221. DOI: 10.1210/jc.2004-0352

[25] Barber KJ, Franklyn JA, McCabe CJ, Khanim FL, Bulmer JN, Whitley GS, et al. The in vitro effects of triiodothyronine on epidermal growth factor-induced trophoblast function. The Journal of Clinical Endocrinology and Metabolism. 2005;**90**:1655-1661. DOI: 10.1210/jc.2004-0785

[26] Kilby MD, Verhaeg J, Gittoes N, Somerset DA, Clark PMS, Franklyn JA. Circulating thyroid hormone concentrations and placental thyroid hormone receptor expression in normal human pregnancy and pregnancy complicated by intrauterine growth restriction (IUGR). The Journal of Clinical Endocrinology and Metabolism. 1998;**83**(8):2964-2971. DOI: 10.1210/jcem.83.8.5002

[27] Thorpe-Beeston JG, Nicolaides K, Snijders JM, Felton CV, McGregor AM. Thyroid function in small for gestational age fetuses. Obstetrics and Gynecology. 1991;**77**:701-706

[28] Redman CW, Sacks GP, Sargent IL. Preeclampsia: An excessive maternal inflammatory response to pregnancy. American Journal of Obstetrics and Gynecology.

1999;**180**:499-506. DOI: 10.1016/S0002-9378(99)70239-5

[29] Benyo DF, Smarason A, Redman CW, Sims C, Conrad KP. Expression of inflammatory cytokines in placentas from women with preeclampsia. The Journal of Clinical Endocrinology and Metabolism. 2001;**86**:2505-2512. DOI: 10.1210/jc.86.6.2505

[30] Parham M, Asgarani F, Bagherzadeh M, Ebrahimi G, Vafaeimanesh J. Thyroid function in pregnant women with gestational diabetes: Is screening necessary? Thyroid Disease in Pregnancy. 2015;**12**:3-7. DOI: 10.4103/0973-0354.147271

[31] Olivieri A, Valensise H, Magnani F, Medda E, DeAngelis S, D'Archivio M, et al. High frequency of antithyroid autoantibodies in pregnant women at increased risk of gestational diabetes mellitus. European Journal of Endocrinology. 2000;**143**:741-747. DOI: 10.1530/eje.0.1430741

[32] Agarwal MM, Dhatt GS, Punnose J, Bishawi B, Zayed R. Thyroid function abnormalities and antithyroid antibody prevalence in pregnant women at high risk for gestational diabetes mellitus. Gynecological Endocrinology. 2006;**22**(5):261-266. DOI: 10.1080/09513590600630470

[33] Ortega-Gonzalez C, Liao-Lo A, Ramirez-Peredo J, Carino N, Lira J, Parra A. Thyroid peroxidase antibodies in Mexican born healthy pregnant women, in women with type 2 or gestational diabetes mellitus, and in their offspring. Endocrine Practice. 2000;**6**:244-248. DOI: 10.4158/EP.6.3.244

[34] Krassas GE, Poppe K, Glinoer D. Thyroid function and human reproductive health. Endocrine Reviews. 2010;**31**:702-755. DOI: 10.1210/er.2009-0041

[35] Casey BM, Dashe JS, Wells CE, McIntire DD, Byrd W, Leveno KJ, et al. Subclinical hypothyroidism and pregnancy outcomes. Obstetrics and Gynecology. 2005;**105**(2):239-245. DOI: 10.1097/01.AOG.0000152345.99421.22

[36] Klein RZ, Haddow JE, Faix JD, Brown RS, Hermos RJ, Pulkkinen A, et al. Prevalence of thyroid deficiency in pregnant women. Clinical Endocrinology. 1991;**35**:41-46. DOI: 10.1111/j.1365-2265.1991.tb03494.x

[37] Allan WC, Haddow JE, Palomaki GE, Williams JR, Mitchell ML, Hermos RJ, et al. Maternal thyroid deficiency and pregnancy complications: Implications for population screening. Journal of Medical Screening. 2000;**7**:127-130

[38] Gharib H, Cobin RH, Dickey RA. Subclinical hypothyroidism during pregnancy: Position statement from the American Association of Clinical Endocrinologists. Endocrine Practice. 1999;**5**(6):367-368

[39] Rao VR, Lakshmi A, Sadhnani MD. Prevalence of hypothyroidism in recurrent pregnancy loss in first trimester. Indian Journal of Medical Sciences. 2008;**62**:357-361. DOI: 10.4103/0019-5359.43122

[40] Stagnaro-Green A, Abalovich M, Alexander E, Azizi F, Mestman J, Negro R, et al. Guidelines of the American Thyroid Association for the Diagnosis and Management of Thyroid Disease During Pregnancy and Postpartum. Thyroid. 2011;**21**:1081-1125. DOI: 10.1089/thy.2011.0087

[41] Balucan FS, Morshed SA, Davies TF. Thyroid autoantibodies in pregnancy: Their role, regulation and clinical relevance. Journal of Thyroid Research. 2013:182472. DOI: 10.1155/2013/182472

[42] Stagnaro-Green A. Thyroid antibodies and miscarriage: Where

are we at a generation later? Journal of Thyroid Research. 2011;**2011**:841949

[43] Mannisto T, Vaarasmaki M, Pouta A, Hartikainnen AL, Ruokonen A, Surcel HM, et al. Thyroid dysfunction and autoantibodies during pregnancy as predictive factors of pregnancy complications and maternal morbidity in later life. The Journal of Clinical Endocrinology and Metabolism. 2010;**95**:1084-1094. DOI: 10.1210/jc.2009-1904

[44] Prummel MF, Wiersinga WM. Thyroid autoimmunity and miscarriage. European Journal of Endocrinology. 2004;**150**(6):751-755

[45] Negro R, Formoso G, Mangieri T, Pezzarossa A, Dazzi D, Hassan H. Levothyroxine treatment in euthyroid pregnant women with autoimmune thyroid disease: Effects on obstetrical complications. The Journal of Clinical Endocrinology and Metabolism. 2006;**91**(7):2587-2591

[46] Bussen S, Steck T. Thyroid antibodies and their relation to antithrombin antibodies, anticardiolipin antibodies and lupus anticoagulant in women with recurrent spontaneous abortions. European Journal of Obstetrics & Gynecology and Reproductive Biology. 1997;**74**:139-143

[47] Glinoer D, Lemone M. Goiter and pregnancy: A new insight into an old problem. Thyroid. 1992;**2**(1):65-70

[48] Bhattacharyya R, Mukherjee K, Das A, Biswas MR, Basunia SR, Mukherjee A. Anti-thyroid peroxidase antibody positivity during early pregnancy is associated with pregnancy complications and maternal morbidity in later life. Journal of Natural Science, Biology and Medicine. 2015;**6**(2):402-405. DOI: 10.4103/0976-9668.160021

[49] Nøhr SB, Jørgensen A, Pedersen KM, Laurberg P. Postpartum thyroid dysfunction in pregnant thyroid peroxidase antibody-positive women living in an area with mild to moderate iodine deficiency: Is iodine supplementation safe? The Journal of Clinical Endocrinology and Metabolism. 2000;**85**(9):3191-3198

[50] Alexander EK, Pearce EN, Brent GA, Brown RS, Chen H, Dosiou C, et al. 2017 Guidelines of the American Thyroid Association for the Diagnosis and Management of Thyroid Disease during pregnancy and the postpartum. Thyroid. 2017;**27**(3):315-389. DOI: 10.1089/thy.2016.0457

[51] Revelli A, Casano S, Piane LD, et al. A retrospective study on IVF outcome in euthyroid patients with anti-thyroid antibodies: Effects of levothyroxine, acetyl-salicylic acid and prednisolone adjuvant treatments. Reproductive Biology and Endocrinology. 2009;**7**:137

[52] Zhong YP, Ying Y, Wu HT, Zhou CQ, Xu YW, Wang Q, et al. Relationship between antithyroid antibody and pregnancy outcome following in vitro fertilization and embryo transfer. International Journal of Medical Sciences. 2012;**9**(2):121-125. DOI: 10.7150/ijms.3467

[53] Bussen S, Steck T, Dietl J. Increased prevalence of thyroid antibodies in euthyroid women with a history of recurrent in-vitro fertilization failure. Human Reproduction. 2000;**15**:545-548

[54] Ghazeeri GS, Kutteh WH. Autoimmune factors in reproductive failure. Current Opinion in Obstetrics & Gynecology. 2001;**13**:287-291

Chapter 3

Mathematical Modeling of Thyroid Size and Hypothyroidism in Hashimoto's Thyroiditis

Balamurugan Pandiyan

Abstract

This chapter is devoted to studying the physiology of the pituitary-thyroid axis and thyroid size in autoimmune thyroiditis via modeling. The pituitary-thyroid axis consists of a feed forward and backward loop in humans, which is responsible for maintaining the body's metabolism. Under a disease situation, the dynamics of the axis becomes more complex and unique among patients. Hashimoto's autoimmune thyroiditis disrupts the normal operation of the axis by slowly destroying the thyroid follicle cells through complex immune mechanisms. So, the size of thyroid and the axis operation are fully, partly, or totally not functional in this disease. Basically, the patient situation in the disease process is unique in describing the diffused goiter and/or a clinical symptom of hashitoxicosis, euthyroidism, subclinical hypothyroidism, or overt hypothyroidism. Using patient-specific modeling, we can predict the hidden dynamics of the natural history of autoimmune thyroiditis and test hypothesis on the operation of axis. In addition, we unfold case studies of three patients from the thyroid literature through the modeling viewpoint and describe their hidden dynamics.

Keywords: Hashimoto's thyroiditis, chronic lymphocytic thyroiditis, goiter, hypothyroidism, patient-specific modeling, pituitary-thyroid axis

1. Introduction

The normal operation of the pituitary-thyroid axis depends on the levels of thyroid stimulating hormone (TSH) and thyroid hormones, triiodothyronine (T3) and thyroxine (T4) [1]. Serum TSH is produced and released by the pituitary gland in response to the low levels of free thyroid hormones in the serum. Circulating TSH in turn stimulates the thyroid to produce and secrete T3 and T4 into the serum. When thyroid hormones reach their highest levels, it inhibits the production of TSH, which describes the normal day to day operation of the pituitary-thyroid axis. The axis is commonly referred as an important negative feedback loop in the endocrine system. The normal function of this loop is essential for the body's metabolic rate—it affects how quickly the cells in our body use the energy stored within itself [2, 3]. For the purpose of this modeling work, we use only serum free T4 for the levels of thyroid hormones as frequently asked to measure in the thyroid clinics for all patients with Hashimoto's autoimmune thyroiditis (see **Figure 1**).

IntechOpen

The normal operation of the axis can be tested and verified clinically via one measurement of TSH and free T4 from the blood serum. Laboratory tests are important in diagnosing conditions of the thyroid gland [2]. The result of the blood test is determined approximately based on the normal reference range of TSH and free T4 is (0.4–4) mU/L and (7–18) pg/mL, respectively as recommended by the American Thyroid Association [2]. As the physiology of the axis is governed by TSH and free T4, the clinical state of the axis has been defined based on these values [3]. Suppose TSH and free T4 levels falls within the normal reference range; the state of the axis is said to be clinically normal. Suppose TSH levels falls above 4 mU/L but free T4 levels falls within the reference range; the state of the axis is said to be clinically subclinical hypothyroidism. Suppose TSH levels are above 4 mU/L and free T4 levels below 7 pg/mL; the state of the axis is said to be clinically hypothyroidism (an underactive thyroid gland). Keeping free T4 levels within the normal reference range is very important [3]. Lower levels of free T4 can cause hypothyroidism that results in several health problems including obesity, joint pain, infertility, slow metabolism, puffy face, constipation, stiffness, dry skin, depression, fatigue and higher heart rate [4].

Hyperthyroidism is another clinical state of the axis, in which free T4 levels stay above 18 pg/mL while the levels of TSH stay below the reference range 0.4 mU/L [5]. This state of the axis occurs when the thyroid gland over produces and secretes the thyroid hormones either in response to chronic TSH stimulation or due to Graves' disease. Transient hyperthyroidism is a phenomenon that refers to the leakage of stored thyroid hormones from the gland, typically called Hashitoxicosis or thyroid burst [6]. It happens due to the Hashimoto's autoimmune thyroiditis. The bursting of thyroid gland can happen at any clinical stage of the patients.

Hashimoto's autoimmune thyroiditis is one of the immune disorders hosted by the thyroid gland [6, 7]. Under this disease process, the thyroid follicular tissue undergoes the slow destruction by the immune system and thereby the thyroid struggles to produce enough hormones for the body's requirement. Currently, the incidence rate of Hashimoto's autoimmune thyroiditis is estimated to be 300–500 cases per 100,000 individuals per year. In this disease, the interaction of the immune system with the thyroid is highly complex involving the cellular and humoral mechanisms. The involvement of humoral mechanism can be verified

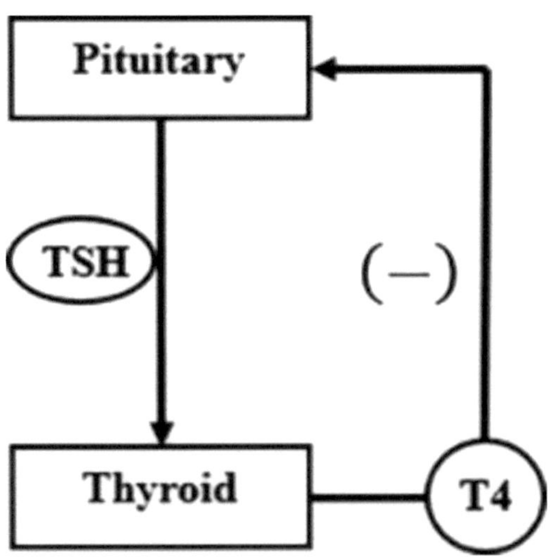

Figure 1.
The pituitary-thyroid axis is shown in this picture. It is commonly referred as a negative-feedback control.

through a simple blood test for anti-thyroid antibody biomarkers. More specifically, the elevated titers of anti-thyroid antibodies, thyroid peroxidase antibodies (TPOAb) and/or thyroglobulin antibodies (TGAb) may indicate the malfunction of the immune system [8]. For simplicity in patient-specific modeling, we choose TPOAb as a biomarker representing the presence of the Hashimoto's autoimmune thyroiditis.

In 1912, Hakaru Hashimoto published the description of four cases of diffused goiter which were showing the signs of infiltration of immune cells and antibodies in the thyroid gland [9]. All these goiters appeared differently from the colloid goiters that occur due to insufficient iodine in-take from the diet. In his time, the idea of autoimmune disease had not been established in the medical literature. He isolated these cases and asked the future clinicians to explore the mechanism of this new form of goiter [10, 11]. In 1936, the description of goiter due to lymphocytic thyroiditis was rediscovered in the United States and was labeled as Hashimoto's thyroiditis. It has been characterized as an organ-specific autoimmune disease and swelling might be the result of the chronic stimulation of the thyroid gland by the serum TSH [12, 13]. Now, scientists have described autoimmune thyroiditis with atrophy, a variance from the original description of Hakaru Hashimoto.

The pituitary gland has no clue about the undergoing immune process in the thyroid gland and does not know how to adapt to the changing environment and the abnormal function of the thyroid [14, 15]. It simply tells the thyroid to keep up with the release of thyroid hormones for its signal. By responding through bulging its size, the poor thyroid gland needs to accomplish the task of producing enough levels of hormones if it could. What initiates the immune process against the thyroid gland? The answer is still largely unknown to the researchers, but they all speculate the immune process might be initiated through a complex combination of the genetic and environmental pollution [15]. Herein, we care about the functional size of thyroid gland as opposed to the exact size of the thyroid gland, which is treated as a hidden compartment [16]. The exact size of the thyroid gland includes the size of the parathyroid glands, the isthmus, capillaries, blood flow and so on whereas the functional size includes the follicular cells that contains thyroglobulin molecules in which hormones are stored. Basically, the functional size of the gland counts the part of the gland that is able to make and secrete hormones; obviously this information is not available in the clinical setting.

A measurement of TPOAb titers is required from the blood test to diagnose autoimmune thyroiditis and afterward, TPOAb titers is not usually measured as its levels not helpful in the treatment. As mentioned above, the axis function is determined from one-time measurement of TSH and free T4, respectively. However, the functional size of the thyroid gland cannot be measured through the laboratory experiments or with any medical tools, which does not exist in practice at least so far. Even if it exists, then it would be very expensive in terms of cost and time. However, the mathematical model can help by telling us the functional size from the clinical measurements of specific patient and from the physiological point of view. Moreover, the functional size of the gland is different for everyone, such as boy's thyroid size versus men's thyroid size or girl's thyroid size versus women's thyroid size and so on. Using the model and the clinical measurements of TSH and free T4, we will determine the initial functional size of the gland for a given patient. Goiter due to this disease occurs more frequently in women than men [17]. Using the model, we describe the diffused goiter as the functional size increases to keep up with the normal production of hormones.

In reality, it is hard to perform experiments on patients in the laboratory setting and collect data to understand the underlying dynamics of the pituitary-thyroid axis in autoimmune problem. Hypothetically speaking, if the experiment is possible, then one needs to consider patients' time, cost, safety, and variability. Two patients with similar characteristics from societies might react to an experiment in an unusual way [18, 19]. The inter and intra variability among patients causes a major problem for treatment and challenges the obtained information from labs. Using the model, we can carry out an experiment for a specific patient and the hidden dynamics of the axis can be investigated at the microscopic level for shorter or longer time-period. In general, the model is implemented through a computer program and the parameters are tuned to a specific patient and then the experiments can be performed with the test hypothesis [20]. Also, we can identify sensitive and insensitive parameters that are responsible for the physiology of the axis under autoimmune thyroiditis, that causes the hypothyroidism and goiter. This is an effective and modern way to explore the complex interaction of the immune system to the thyroid and its consequence on the negative feedback loop [21, 22].

The hormone TSH has a half-life of 1 hour in serum on the average scale. Similarly, the hormone free T4 has a half-life of 7 days in serum on average, the thyroid per-oxidase antibodies (TPOAb) has a half-life of 24 hours in serum on average and the half-life of functional size of the thyroid gland is not known and probably varies among individuals. Several time scales have been involved in the disease process. Based on the fundamental principle of rate laws, the model will be developed here to predict the history of patient-specific dynamics of the axis and thyroid size in autoimmune thyroiditis [23–25]. The model can unfold the consequences of the presence of antibodies titers in the blood. Basically, it can replace humans but mimics the system that provides convenience and flexibility for scientists to run experiments on the computer. Information obtained through the dynamics might be useful in treating patients and improving the accuracy of the levothyroxine treatment [26]. For instance, the levothyroxine drug can be targeted and administered to the specific patient so that the levels of TSH and free T4 maintained within the normal reference range, which in turn can avoid other health problems.

The remaining of this chapter is divided into three main sections. Section 2 introduces the development and construction of a coupled model describing the interactions of two subsystems (the axis and humoral immune system) and reduces the coupled model based on the physiological assumptions. Section 3 analyzes the solutions of the reduced model qualitatively and numerically for various parameter values. Section 4 describes the case studies of three patients, validity of the model and provides the conclusion of this work.

2. Model outline

The model is constructed as a system of four ordinary differential equations based on the following known physiological assumptions [20, 21].

2.1 Assumptions

1. The pituitary gland is diseased free, so the feed forward loop is intact.

2. Total TSH receptors concentration does not change during Hashimoto's autoimmune thyroiditis.

3. Serum TSH stimulates the growth of functional thyroid and the production and secretion of thyroid hormones.

4. The humoral immune system uses serum TPOAb to attack the thyroid and those titers can be used as a biomarker for the level of the anti-thyroid immune activity.

5. The patient does not demonstrate central or peripheral resistance to thyroid hormone.

6. Serum free T4 have much slower dynamics in the disease process compared to serum TSH, serum TPOAb and the functional size of the gland.

We denote $x(t), y(t)$ and $w(t)$ to represent the concentrations of serum TSH (mU/L), serum free T4 (pg/mL) and serum TPOAb (U/mL), respectively. We let $z(t)$ represent the functional size of the gland. According to the fundamental principle of rate laws, the rate of change of concentration of TSH over time t is the secretion rate from the pituitary gland minus the elimination rate of TSH via kidney through the unspecified mechanism. The rate of change of concentration of free T4 over time t is the secretion rate of free T4 from the thyroid minus the elimination rate of free T4 via kidney through unspecified mechanism. Similarly, the rate of change of concentration of TPOAb over time t is the production rate due to the abnormal interaction thyroid gland and immune system minus the elimination rate of TPOAb via kidney through unspecified mechanism. Finally, the rate of change of the functional size of thyroid gland over time t is the growth rate minus the destruction rate of the gland.

Next, we write a coupled model that represents the interaction of two subsystems: the negative feedback loop and the humoral immune system.

$$\frac{dx}{dt} = k_1 - \frac{k_1 y(t)}{k_a + y(t)} - k_2 x(t), \qquad x(0) = x_0 \tag{1}$$

$$\frac{dy}{dt} = \frac{k_3 z(t) x(t)}{k_d + x(t)} - k_4 y(t), \qquad y(0) = y_0 \tag{2}$$

$$\frac{dz}{dt} = k_5 \left(\frac{x(t)}{z(t)} - N \right) - k_6 z(t) w(t) \qquad z(0) = z_0 \tag{3}$$

$$\frac{dw}{dt} = k_7 z(t) w(t) - k_8 w(t) \qquad w(0) = w_0 \tag{4}$$

where $x(t) \geq 0, y(t) \geq 0, z(t) > 0$ and $w(t) \geq 0$. The normal average value for each state variable is given in **Table 1**. The model has 11 positive parameters unchanged over time, in which each parameter has a unique physiological meaning and their corresponding values listed in **Table 2**. The model (1)–(4) captured the dynamics of two subsystems coupled through the functional size of the thyroid gland. Using assumption (8) that serum free T4 has much slower dynamics compared to serum

Name	Normal value	Normal range	Source	Unit
$x(t)$	1	$0.4 - (2.5 - 4)$	Literature [2]	mU/L
$y(t)$	13	$7 - 18$	Literature [2]	pg/mL
$z(t)$	0.015	$0.005 - 0.125$	Literature [16]	L
$w(t)$	0	$0 - <200$	Dataset	U/mL

Table 1.
Variable names, normal values, ranges, sources and units.

Name	Normal value	Normal range	Source	Unit
k_1	5000	> 4000	Literature [27]	mU/L day
k_2	16.6	N/A	Literature [3]	1/day
k_3	90.11	4 – 257	Simulation	Pg/mL L day
k_4	0.099021	N/A	Literature [3]	1/day
k_5	1	N/A	Simulation	L^3/mU day
k_6	1	N/A	Simulation	mL/U day
k_8	0.035	N/A	Literature [28]	1/day
k_a	0.043	0.02 – 0.06	Calculation	pg/mL
k_d	0.05	N/A	Simulation	mU/L^2

Table 2.
Parameter names, normal values, ranges, sources and units.

TSH, serum TPOAb and the functional size of the thyroid gland, we can take $dy/dt = 0$ and obtain a reduced model consisting of three differential equations and one algebraic equation:

$$\frac{dx}{dt} = \frac{k_1 k_4 k_a (k_d + x(t))}{k_4 k_a k_d + k_4 k_a x(t) + k_3 z(t) x(t)} - k_2 x(t), \qquad x(0) = x_0 \tag{5}$$

$$z = \frac{k_4 y (k_d + x)}{k_3 x} = f(x, y) \tag{6}$$

Using (Eq. (6)), the functional size can be determined for patients if a result of TSH (x) and free T4 (y) value is known from the blood test, which in turn can be used as an initial condition on (Eq. (3)) for the model simulation. The graph of (Eq. (6)) is shown on the **Figure 2**, which illustrates the functional size of thyroid gland in terms of varying TSH and free T4 values. Using the reduced

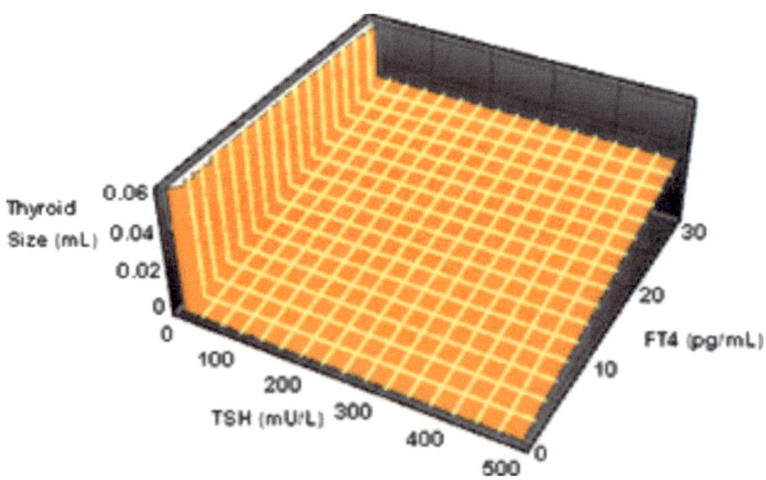

Figure 2.
The functional size of the thyroid gland can be calculated from the graph of this function of TSH and free T4.

model, we can describe the clinical progression of overt hypothyroidism and thyroid size such as goiter and atrophy.

3. Model analysis

As a first step in the process of analyzing the model, we solve for steady states of the reduced model (Eqs. (3)–(5)) from the following equations:

$$\frac{k_1 k_4 k_a (k_d + x)}{k_4 k_a k_d + k_4 k_a x + k_3 z x} - k_2 x = 0$$

$$k_5\left(\frac{x}{z} - N\right) - k_6 z w = 0$$

$$k_7 z w - k_8 w = 0$$

which leads to diseased-free and diseased steady state solutions besides the initial condition. The first steady state (diseased-free) denoted as (z_1, w_1, x_1) where $z_1 = x_1/N, w_1 = 0$ and the value of x_1 is given by the cubic equation:

$$a_1 {x_1}^3 + a_2 {x_1}^2 + a_3 x_1 + a_4 = 0 \quad (7)$$

where

$$a_1 = \frac{k_2 k_3}{N} > 0$$

$$a_2 = k_2 k_4 k_a > 0$$

$$a_3 = k_4 k_a (k_d k_2 - k_1) < 0 \text{ since } k_1 > k_d k_2$$

$$a_4 = -k_4 k_a k_1 k_d < 0$$

By Descarte's rule of signs, Eq. (7) has one positive real solution, so the reduced model has diseased-free state in the positive octant for the system parameters. In fact, this steady state solution lives on the surface of the function $z = f(x, y)$ given by Eq. (6). The operation of the pituitary-thyroid axis is healthy and fully functional in the presence of diseased-free steady state solution.

Next, the second steady state is the diseased state solution denoted as (z_2, w_2, x_2) where

$$z_2 = \frac{k_8}{k_7}$$

$$w_2 = \frac{k_7 k_5}{k_6 k_8}\left(\frac{k_7 x_2}{k_8} - N\right)$$

and the value x_2 is given by the quadratic equation:

$$b_1 {x_2}^2 + b_2 x_2 + b_3 = 0 \quad (8)$$

where

$$b_1 = \left(k_2 k_4 k_a + \frac{k_2 k_3 k_8}{k_7}\right) > 0$$

$$b_2 = k_4 k_a (k_d k_2 - k_1) < 0 \text{ since } k_1 > k_d k_2$$

$$b_3 = -k_4 k_a k_1 k_d < 0$$

By Descarte's rule of signs, Eq. (8) has one positive real solution when $x_2 > \frac{Nk_8}{k_7}$ so the reduced model has diseased state in the positive octant for the system parameters.

Remark: When $N = k_7 x_2 / k_8$, the second steady state (diseased state) of the system (Eqs. (3)–(5)) has $w_2 = 0$. So, it must coincide with the first steady state (diseased-free state) in the positive quadrant if

$$N = \frac{k_7 x_2}{k_8} = \frac{k_7 x_1}{k_8}$$

3.1 Definition: bifurcation parameter

We let N^* be the unique value of N, where

$$N^* = \frac{k_7 x_0}{k_8} = \frac{k_7 x_2}{k_8} = \frac{k_7 x_1}{k_8}$$

the system undergoes a bifurcation. We call N^* is a bifurcation value of the system (Eqs. (3)–(5)) and N is the bifurcation parameter. We can take the initial state of the system at where the diseased-free and diseased steady states merge together. Using this definition, we can also calculate the parameter k_7 (say $k_7{}^*$) provided the values of k_8 and x_0 is known.

3.2 Equation of tangent plane

We first define the level surface (S) through a function of three variables from Eq. (6) as

$$g(x(t), y(t), z(t)) = \frac{k_4 y(t)(k_d + x(t))}{k_3 x(t)} - z(t) = 0 \tag{9}$$

The normal surface vector $\vec{n}$ can be calculated from the gradient of this function

$$\vec{n} = \langle \frac{\partial g}{\partial x}, \frac{\partial g}{\partial y}, \frac{\partial g}{\partial z} \rangle$$

In particular, the normal vector of the surface S at initial state $P(x_0, y_0, z_0)$ is a vector perpendicular to the tangent plane of S at P is given by

$$\vec{n} = \langle \frac{-k_4 k_d y_0}{k_3 x_0{}^2}, \left(\frac{k_4 k_d}{k_3 x_0} + \frac{k_4}{k_3}\right), -1 \rangle$$

The equation of the tangent plane at point $P(x_0, y_0, z_0)$ is given by

$$ax + by + cz = d$$

where

$$a = \frac{-k_4 k_d y_0}{k_3 x_0{}^2}, b = \left(\frac{k_4 k_d}{k_3 x_0} + \frac{k_4}{k_3}\right), c = -1 \wedge$$

$$d = ax_0 + by_0 + cz_0$$

Next, we take the implicit differentiation of Eq. (9) with respect to time t and substituting the initial point $P(x_0, y_0, z_0, w_0)$, which results in the following equation for N:

$$\left(\frac{\partial g}{\partial x}\bullet\frac{dx}{dt}+\frac{\partial g}{\partial y}\bullet\frac{dy}{dt}+\frac{\partial g}{\partial z}\bullet\frac{dz}{dt}\right)_P=0$$

$$N=\frac{-k_4y_0(-k_1k_ak_d-x_0(-k_2k_d+k_4(k_d+x_0))(k_a+y_0))}{k_5k_3x_0^2(k_a+y_0)}+\frac{x_0}{z_0}-\frac{(k_4+k_6w_0)z_0}{k_5} \tag{10}$$

Notice that N is independent of the parameters k_7 and k_8. So, we can use this value of N as N^*. This threshold value can be uniquely determined for every patient based on their initial blood test results and if we know other parameters $k_1, k_2, k_3, k_4, k_5, k_6, k_a$ and k_d. We have estimated the values of all other parameters from the literature or through calculation (see **Table 2**).

3.3 Linear stability

As the bifurcation parameter N varies from the threshold value $N^* = k_7x_0/k_8$, the number of the steady states changes, and its behavior near the steady states (linear stability) changes as well. Moreover, as the bifurcation parameter varies, the appearance and disappearance of steady states can be seen on the tangent plane at the initial state of the function $z = f(x, y)$. For this system (Eqs. (3)–(5)), there are three cases, namely when $N < N^*$, $N = N^*$ and $N > N^*$. **Figure 3** illustrates a nice overview of how the solutions become stable and unstable as parameter N changes from 0 to 300.

Case 1: $N < N^*$

When $N < N^*$, the system (Eqs. (3)–(5)) has two steady states, which undergoes a saddle-node bifurcation—disappearance of the saddle diseased state. One can

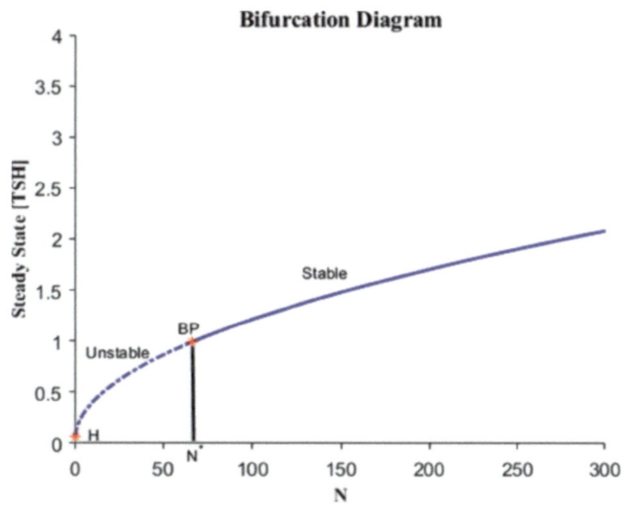

Figure 3.
The bifurcation diagram shows the steady state values of TSH as the parameter N varies from 0 to 300. BP means the branch or bifurcation point where another equilibrium curve passes through and the system switches its stability. The parameter value of N at BP is 66.7. H is a neutral saddle, but not the bifurcation point for the equilibrium curve. At H, there is a homoclinic orbit for the system.

imagine if we start the system from the initial steady state, which splits into the diseased-free and diseased state. The disease state is asymptotically stable which means all its eigenvalues are purely negative real. However, the diseased-free state is saddle because two of its eigenvalues are positive real and one of its eigenvalues is a negative real. See [22] for proof of the stability of the diseased-free and diseased steady state.

As the value of N decreases from the threshold value and when it is close to zero, there exists a homoclinic orbit associated at the initial state which forms the boundary for the asymptomatically stable interior diseased state. The orbit captures the hidden dynamics of the diffused goiter and hashitoxicosis (see **Figures 4** and 5).

Case 2: $N = N^*$

When $N = N^*$, the system (Eqs. (3)–(5)) has one steady state (diseased-free), which is asymptotically stable. Since there is only one steady state in the system, the operation of the pituitary-thyroid axis in the presence of anti-thyroid peroxidase

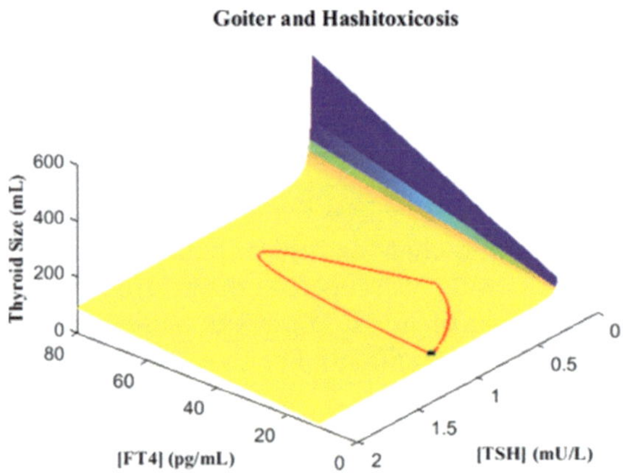

Figure 4.
When the value of N = 10 and $k_7 = 2.3345$, the hidden dynamics of the axis and the thyroid size reveal hashitoxicosis and goiter. The model simulation is performed for 2 years from the initial state: TSH = 1 mU/L, free T4 = 13 pg/mL, and thyroid size = 0.015 mL and TPOAb = 10 U/mL.

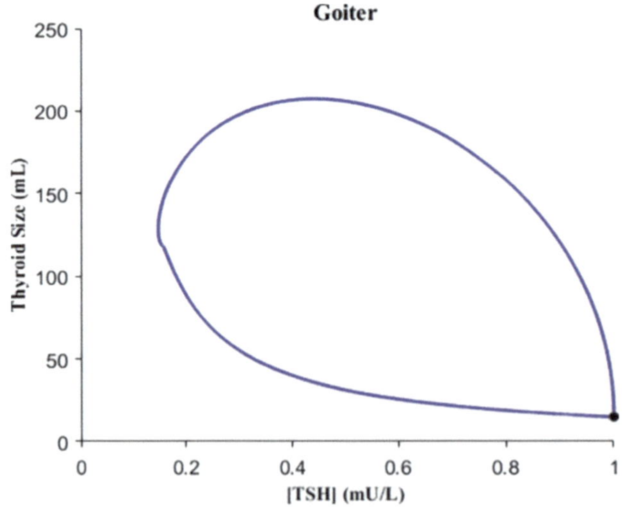

Figure 5.
When N = 0.01 and $k_7 = 2.3345$, the hidden dynamics of the thyroid size capture the development of goiter and return to normal size.

antibodies can be tested. The numerical simulation of the model shows TPOAb slowly approaches zero as time increases over months (see **Figure 6**).

Case 3: $N > N^*$

When $N > N^*$, the system (Eqs. (3)–(5)) has one steady state (diseased-free), which is asymptotically stable. As the value of N increases beyond the threshold value, the diseased free state is moving on the function $z = f(x, y)$ describing the progression of thyroid size and the function of the axis. One can imagine if we start the system from the initial state of normal thyroid size, then the system may approach goiter or atrophy depending upon the parameter value of N while keeping other parameters fixed. On the other hand, varying the parameter k_7, the clinical

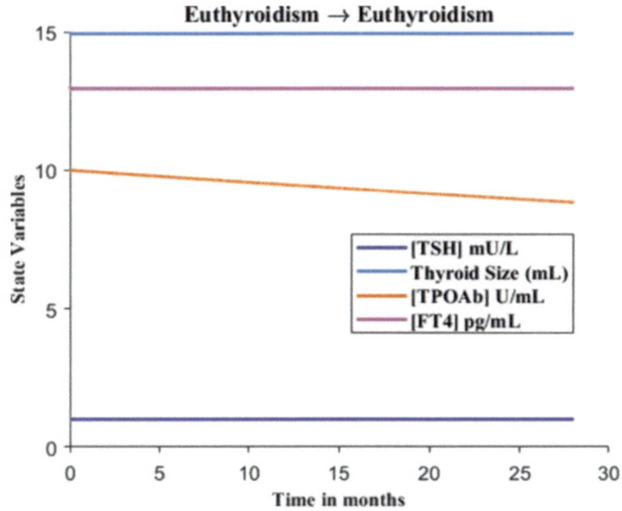

Figure 6.
The parameter value is set to $N = 66.7, k_7 = 2.3345$ and the initial state is at euthyroidism (1, 0.015, 10). The levels of anti-thyroid peroxidase decrease slowly whereas TSH and the functional thyroid size remains unchanged over time, which indicates the normal operation of the axis with fully functional thyroid size.

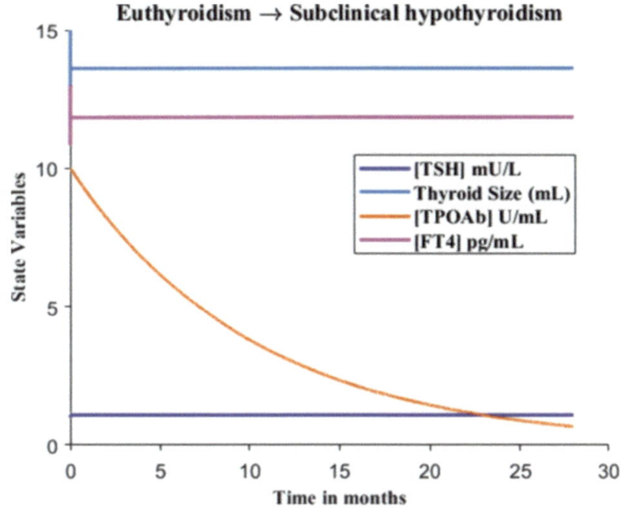

Figure 7.
Clinical progression from euthyroidism to mild subclinical hypothyroidism when $N = 80, k_7 = 2.3345$ with initial state (1, 0.015, 10).

mechanisms euthyroidism → subclinical hypothyroidism → overt hypothyroidism can be explained while keeping N fixed [20]. See **Figure 7** that shows the clinical progression of subclinical hypothyroidism and thyroid size.

3.4 Exploration of parameter curve

Suppose that an individual is diagnosed with Hashimoto's autoimmune thyroiditis; we can use the reduced model to explain the physical and clinical symptoms occurring for this individual in the course of this disease. Having this disease means everyone has a unique behavior and knowing that may be very helpful in managing the course. In fact, certain parameter values in the reduced model are responsible for the uniqueness in patient behavior. More specifically, we have identified through the stability analysis that the parameter N can explain the size of the thyroid (goiter, normal or atrophy) whereas k_7 can explain the clinical progression of the disease [21, 22]. Putting these two parameters together, one can test the hypothesis on the patients' symptoms. See **Figure 8** that shows the parameter curve in terms of N and k_7 that is responsible for different thyroid size and clinical conditions.

Suppose a patient's information is given; then a threshold $\left(k_7^*, N^*\right)$ can be found for the patient using Eq. (10) and the definition of the bifurcation parameter. If another information is available in the future, then another threshold can be obtained. To be exact, the threshold is an ordered pair found on the curve given by the bifurcation definition of parameter (see **Figure 8**). To simulate physical and clinical symptoms, we take two test ordered pairs from the parameter curve below and above the threshold $\left(k_7^*, N^*\right) = 2.3345, 66.7)$ while other parameters came from **Table 2**. With the first test point for $(k_7, N) = (0.9904, 12.65)$, we simulated the model for a day and found the symptoms of the disease are hashitoxicosis and goiter (see **Figure 9**). Similarly, by keeping the second test point as (5.8, 397.9), the one-day simulation showed mild atrophy and overt hypothyroidism (see **Figure 10**). Finally, by keeping the third test point away from the curve as (4.5, 150), the one-day simulation showed subclinical hypothyroidism and normal size of the thyroid (**Figure 11**).

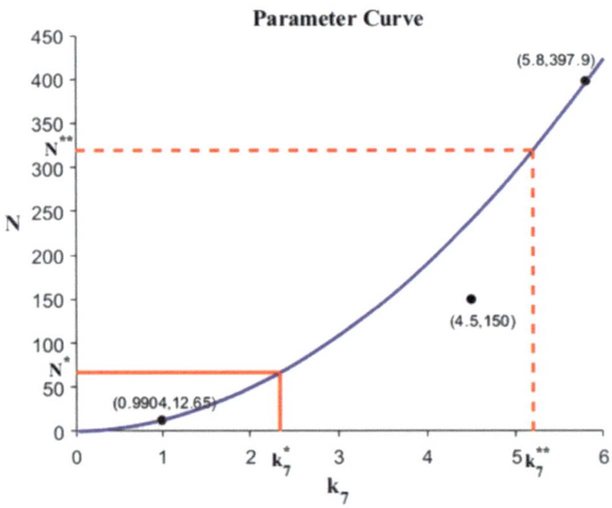

Figure 8.
The sample parameter curve of a Hashimoto's patient is shown here. The hypothesis testing can be done for different k_7 and N values from the curve.

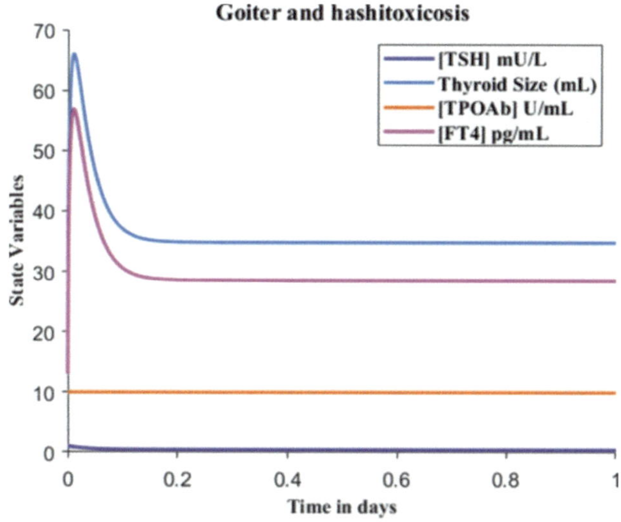

Figure 9.
The result of physical and clinical symptoms is goiter and hashitoxicosis when test values $N = 12.65$ and $k_7 = 0.9904$ are taken from the parameter curve.

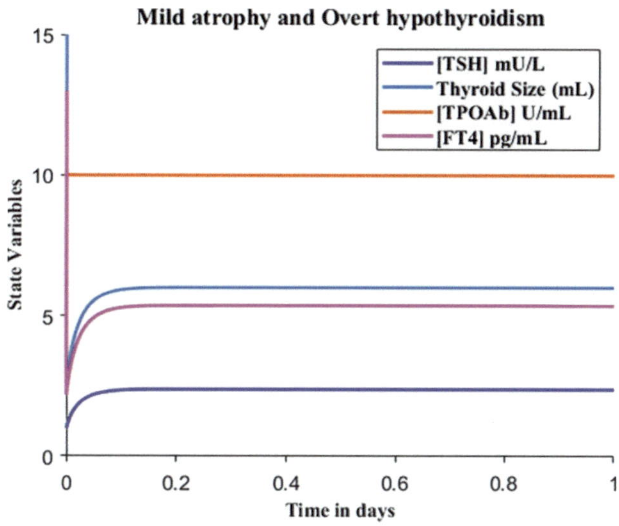

Figure 10.
The result of physical and clinical symptoms is mild atrophy and overt hypothyroidism, when test values $N = 397.9$ and $k_7 = 5.8$ are taken from the curve.

4. Case studies of three patients

Using patients' information from the peer-reviewed published article, we will predict patients' natural history of the disease. More precisely, the reduced model can describe thyroid size and clinical progression from euthyroidism to subclinical or overt hypothyroidism for each patient given below. These patients' information was provided by Salvatore Benvenga originally and were already published in the article [21]. The data consists of TSH, free T4 and TPOAb information whose normal reference ranges are (0.4–2.5) mU/L, (7–18) pg./mL and (0–200) U/mL, respectively. Using Eq. (6) and data, we have computed the functional size of the

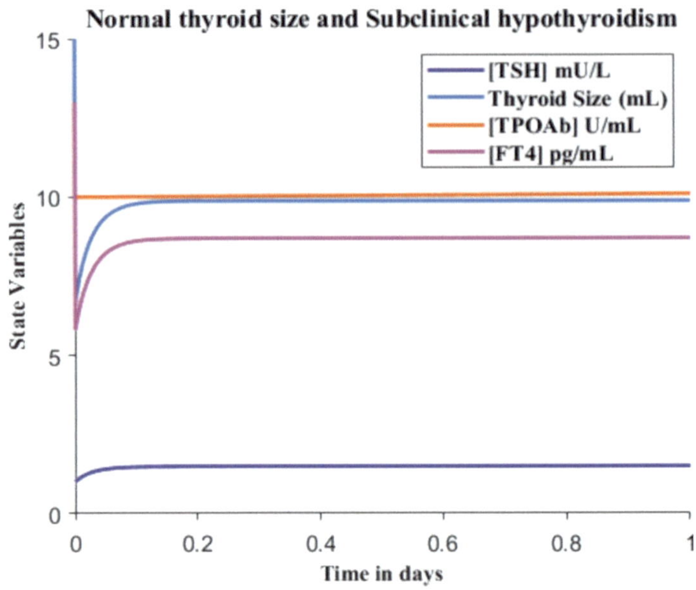

Figure 11.
The result of physical and clinical symptoms are normal thyroid size and subclinical hypothyroidism, when test values of $N = 4.5$ and $k_7 = 150$ are not taken from the curve.

Time (months)	TSH (mU/L)	FT4 (pg/mL)	TPOAb (U/mL)	Thyroid size (mL)	N^*	k_7^*
0	0.8282	13.5	50	15.73	51.865	2.1918
8	0.93	13	55	15.1	60.952	2.2939
30	1.178	11.8	159	13.5	84.998	2.5254

Table 3.
Patient 1 information.

Time (months)	TSH (mU/L)	FT4 (pg/mL)	TPOAb (U/mL)	Thyroid size (mL)	N^*	k_7^*
0	1.54	11.78	3810	13.37	64.301	1.4614
31	1.57	12.36	1310	14.02	93.662	2.088
39	1.54	11.97	1480	13.58	93.294	2.1203

Table 4.
Patient 2 information.

Time (months)	TSH (mU/L)	FT4 (pg/mL)	TPOAb (U/mL)	Thyroid size (mL)	N^*	k_7^*
0	1.46	15.16	164	17.23	81.908	1.9635
2	1.56	13.74	153	15.58	97.724	2.1925
3	1.85	13.09	191	14.77	122.4	2.3157
5	2.06	11.67	482	13.14	150.5	2.557
22	4.61	10.47	773	11.63	387.39	2.9411
39	5.04	7.63	537	8.467	590.65	4.1018

Table 5.
Patient 3 information.

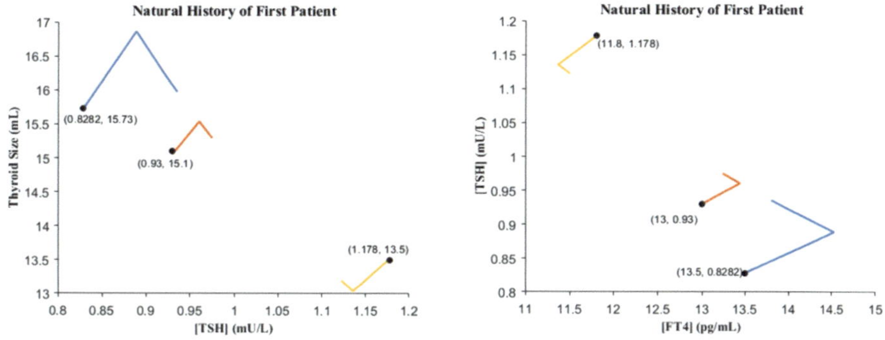

Figure 12.
Three courses of the natural history of the disease is shown here for patient 1. Patient 1 visited the clinic three times and was not required any treatment based on their TSH and free T4 values. The model is simulated for 10 years in which the first course of disease shows thyroid size started with mild goiter and then returned to normal.

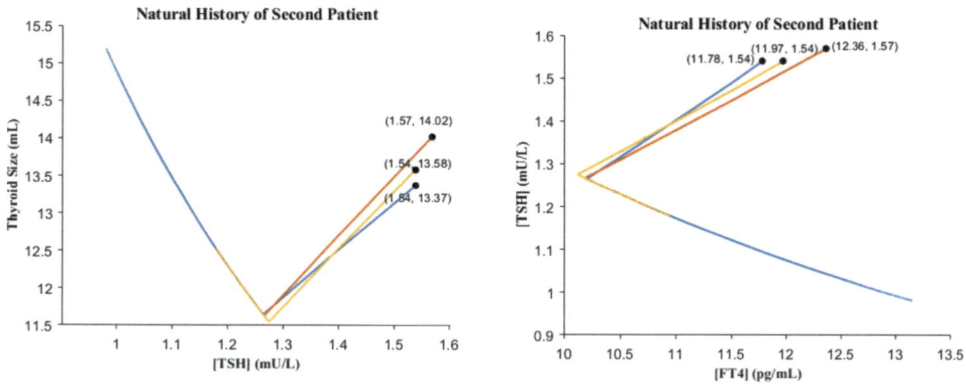

Figure 13.
Three courses of the disease is shown here for the second patient. This patient visited the clinic three times and was not required treatment based on their TSH and free T4 measurements. The model is simulated for 1 year to observe the hidden dynamics. The course of the disease showed patient had developed subclinical hypothyroidism with normal thyroid size.

thyroid gland. Using Eq. (10), data and the bifurcation definition, we have computed N and k_7 for all patients given below (see **Tables 3–5**).

Assuming all patients had diseased-free state (1, 13, 0.015, 0) at some point, the data provides us the diseased state from which one can back trace the physical and clinical conditions caused by the disease and experienced by the patients. We have taken three untreated patients with a known biomarker for the presence of the autoimmune thyroiditis. Patients 1 and 2 visited the clinic three times whereas patient 3 visited the clinic six times due to mild goiter or other symptoms. We do not have any information about their thyroid sizes in the data.

In **Table 3**, the clinical measurements, the functional thyroid size and parameters are listed for patient 1 which form the diseased states. The model simulation started from each diseased state for 10 years to back trace the natural symptoms of patient 1 due to autoimmune thyroiditis. The course of disease revealed thyroid size changes from mild goiter to normal while the function of axis remained normal (see **Figure 12**). In **Table 4**, the clinical measurements, the functional thyroid size and parameters are listed for patient 2. The model simulation is done for 1 year to back trace the symptoms from the course of the disease. The first disease course revealed a development of subclinical hypothyroidism with normal functional thyroid size (see **Figure 13**). Similarly, patient 3 diseased states are found in **Table 5**. The model simulation is done only for 2 days to capture the early course of the disease.

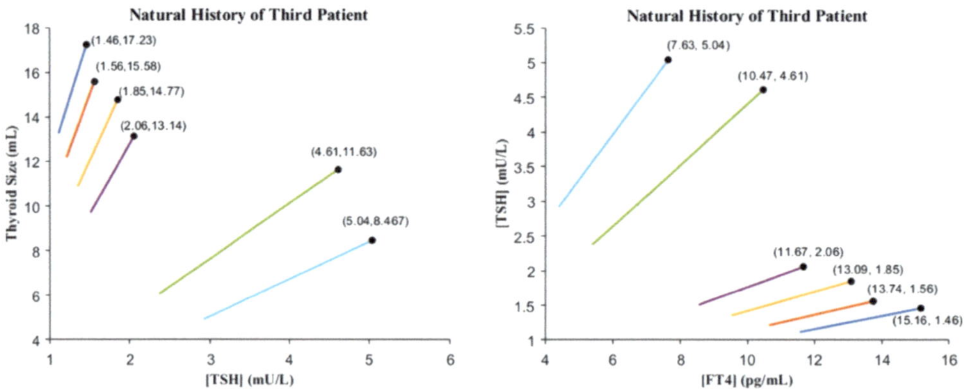

Figure 14.
Six courses of the disease has been shown here for the third patient. This patient visited the clinic six times and was not required any treatment based on their TSH and free T4 measurement. The model is intentionally simulated for 2 days to capture the early dynamics of the patient. The model simulation shows this patient had developed both clinical and physical symptoms at different points in time.

Surprising results are seen in the early course of the disease (see **Figure 14**). This patient had developed both clinical and physical symptoms at different points in time. In particular, the first course shows mild goiter and mild hashitoxicosis whereas the sixth course shows the overt hypothyroidism and mild atrophy.

5. Conclusion

The human body is made up of so many subsystems such as the pituitary-thyroid axis and the immune system. These subsystems do not disrupt the function of each other in healthy people. A function of the pituitary-thyroid axis is to secrete the appropriate levels of thyroid hormones and take care of body's metabolism whereas the function of the immune system is to protect the body's organs such as the thyroid gland and remove foreign substances that try to invade the organs. Hashimoto discovered the abnormal interaction of the immune system to the thyroid gland, which resulted in the disruption of the physiology of the axis. Later this diseased condition has been named as Hashimoto's autoimmune thyroiditis. Hashimoto noticed the destruction of thyroid follicular cells through physical and clinical symptoms in four middle aged female patients.

A keystone of the functional thyroid gland is the follicular cells, which die due to the aggressive and destructive attack by the immune system. Hashimoto patients discovered the disease sometimes by themselves due to discomfort in the neck (small goiter) or accidentally during annual checkup by the family physicians. Consequences of Hashimoto disease can be classified into physical and clinical symptoms at various stages of the disease. Both types of symptoms occur in a sequential manner from one extreme to another. More precisely, the physical symptom runs from goiter → atrophy whereas the clinical symptom runs from hashitoxicosis → overt hypothyroidism. In order to describe these symptoms mathematically, we chose four state variables namely the size of functional thyroid gland to describe the physical symptom, TSH and free T4 to describe the clinical symptoms and thyroid peroxidase antibodies as a representative for the presence of Hashimoto disease. Modeling the disruption of the axis through a coupled model is the key to unlock the hidden dynamics experienced by the patients. The hidden dynamics can be seen in patients through physical and clinical symptoms.

The literature description of Hashimoto disease begins with a gradual swelling of the thyroid gland and development of mild clinical condition, euthyroidism or subclinical hypothyroidism and subsequent gradual progression of overt hypothyroidism. Small goiter and hashitoxicosis are the very early stages of the disease and typically go untreated and hidden in the view of patients and physicians. Overt hypothyroidism is the irreversible end clinical state (where levothyroxine treatment is needed) whereas atrophy is irreversible end physical state of the disease. Basically, the mechanism involved in the progression of the disease is unique and sequential. For instance, some patients may have the disease course of goiter and euthyroidism, some may have goiter and the clinical progression euthyroidism → subclinical hypothyroidism and some patients may have gradual progression from normal thyroid size to atrophy and euthyroidism to overt hypothyroidism.

Herein, we have developed and used patient-specific model to describe all possible mechanisms involved in the autoimmune thyroiditis. This can be achieved using two parameters $\boldsymbol{N}$ and $\boldsymbol{k}_7$. To be precise, the parameter $\boldsymbol{N}$ and $\boldsymbol{k}_7$ can trace the thyroid size and clinical progression. We validated the model with three patients' data by describing their natural history of the disease.

Acknowledgements

I would like to dedicate this chapter to Dr. Stephen J. Merrill for his guidance on mathematical modeling of Hashimoto's autoimmune thyroiditis.

Conflict of interest

We declare there is no conflict of interest on this chapter.

Notes/thanks/other declarations

I would like to thank Dr. Salvatore Benvenga for providing Hashimoto's patients data for the modeling work.

Author details

Balamurugan Pandiyan
University of Wisconsin, Whitewater, WI, USA

*Address all correspondence to: pandiyab@uww.edu

References

[1] Andersen S, Pedersen KM, Bruun NH, Laurberg P. Narrow individual variations in serum T4 and T3 in normal subjects: A clue to the understanding of subclinical thyroid disease. The Journal of Clinical Endocrinology and Metabolism. 2002; **87**(3):1068-1072

[2] Baloch Z, Carayon P, Conte-Devolx B, Demers LM, Feldt-Rasmussen U, Henry JF, et al. Laboratory medicine practice guidelines. Laboratory support for the diagnosis and monitoring of thyroid disease. Thyroid: Official Journal of the American Thyroid Association. 2003;**13**(1):3

[3] Braverman LE, Cooper D. Werner & Ingbar's the Thyroid: A Fundamental and Clinical Text. Philadelphia, PA, USA: Lippincott Williams & Wilkins; 2012

[4] Woolner LB, McConahey WM, Beahrs OH. Struma lymphomatosa (Hashimoto's thyroiditis) and related thyroidal disorders. The Journal of Clinical Endocrinology and Metabolism. 1959;**19**(1):53-83

[5] Woolf PD. Transient painless thyroiditis with hyperthyroidism: A variant of lymphocytic thyroiditis? Endocrine Reviews. 1980;**1**(4):411-420

[6] Kirsten D. The thyroid gland: Physiology and pathophysiology. Neonatal Network. 2000;**19**(8):11-26

[7] Burek CL, Talor MV. Environmental triggers of autoimmune thyroiditis. Journal of Autoimmunity. 2009;**33**(3-4): 183-189

[8] Dayan CM, Daniels GH. Chronic autoimmune thyroiditis. New England Journal of Medicine. 1996;**335**(2):99-107

[9] Hashimoto H. Zur kenntniss der lymphomatosen veranderung der Schilddruse (Struma lymphomatosa). Langenbecks archiv fur klinische chirurgie. 1912;**97**:219-248

[10] Caturegli P, De Remigis A, Rose NR. Hashimoto thyroiditis: Clinical and diagnostic criteria. Autoimmunity Reviews. 2014;**13**(4-5):391-397

[11] Chistiakov DA. Immunogenetics of Hashimoto's thyroiditis. Journal of Autoimmune Diseases. 2005;**2**(1):1

[12] Dunning EJ. Struma lymphomatosa: A report of three cases in one family. The Journal of Clinical Endocrinology and Metabolism. 1959;**19**(9):1121-1125

[13] Fisher DA, Oddie TH, Johnson DE, Nelson JC. The diagnosis of Hashimoto's thyroiditis. The Journal of Clinical Endocrinology and Metabolism. 1975; **40**(5):795-801

[14] Gardner DG, Shoback D, Greenspan FS. Greenspan's Basic & Clinical Endocrinology. New York, NY, USA: McGraw-Hill Medical; 2007

[15] Guarneri F, Benvenga S. Environmental factors and genetic background that interact to cause autoimmune thyroid disease. Current Opinion in Endocrinology, Diabetes and Obesity. 2007;**14**(5):398-409

[16] Carlé A, Pedersen IB, Knudsen N, Perrild H, Ovesen L, Jørgensen T, et al. Thyroid volume in hypothyroidism due to autoimmune disease follows a unimodal distribution: Evidence against primary thyroid atrophy and autoimmune thyroiditis being distinct diseases. The Journal of Clinical Endocrinology and Metabolism. 2009; **94**(3):833-839

[17] Gribetz D, Talbot NB, Crawford JD. Goiter due to lymphocytic thyroiditis (Hashimoto's Struma) its occurrence in preadolescent and adolescent girls.

New England Journal of Medicine. 1954; **250**(13):555-557

[18] Harsch IA, Hahn EG, Strobel D. Hashitoxicosis—Three cases and a review of the literature. European Journal of Endocrinology. 2008;**4**(1): 70-72

[19] Humbert JR, Gotlin RW, Hostetter GL, Sherrill JG, Silver HK. Lymphocytic (auto-immune, Hashimoto's) thyroiditis. Presentation of an unusual case with subacute onset in a 14-year-old girl. Archives of Disease in Childhood. 1968;**43**(227):80

[20] Pandiyan B. Mathematical modeling and dynamical analysis of the operation of the hypothalamus-pituitary-thyroid (HPT) axis in autoimmune (Hashimoto's) thyroiditis [thesis]. Milwaukee, Wisconsin: Marquette University; 2011

[21] Pandiyan B, Merrill SJ, Benvenga S. A patient-specific model of the negative-feedback control of the hypothalamus-pituitary-thyroid (HPT) axis in autoimmune (Hashimoto's) thyroiditis. Mathematical Medicine and Biology: A Journal of the IMA. 2013; **31**(3):226-258

[22] Pandiyan B, Merrill SJ, Benvenga S. A homoclinic orbit in a patient-specific model of Hashimoto's thyroiditis. Differential Equations and Dynamical Systems. 2016:1-8. DOI: 10.1007/s12591-016-0335-5

[23] Nabhan ZM, Kreher NC, Eugster EA. Hashitoxicosis in children: Clinical features and natural history. The Journal of Pediatrics. 2005;**146**(4): 533-536

[24] Volpé R. Autoimmune thyroid diseases. In: Diseases of the Thyroid. Totowa, NJ: Humana Press; 1997. pp. 125-154

[25] Tunbridge WM, Brewis M, French JM, Appleton D, Bird T, Clark F, et al. Natural history of autoimmune thyroiditis. British Medical Journal (Clinical Research Ed.). 1981; **282**(6260):258-262

[26] Schmidt M, Voell M, Rahlff I, Dietlein M, Kobe C, Faust M, et al. Long-term follow-up of antithyroid peroxidase antibodies in patients with chronic autoimmune thyroiditis (Hashimoto's thyroiditis) treated with levothyroxine. Thyroid. 2008;**18**(7): 755-760

[27] Faglia G, Beck-Peccoz P, Piscitelli G, Medri G. Inappropriate secretion of thyrotropin by the pituitary. Hormone Research in Pædiatrics. 1987;**26**(1-4): 79-99

[28] Fröhlich E, Wahl R. Thyroid autoimmunity: Role of anti-thyroid antibodies in thyroid and extra-thyroidal diseases. Frontiers in Immunology. 2017;**8**:521

Chapter 4

Hyperthyroidism

Rushikesh Maheshwari

Abstract

Excess level of thyroid hormones in blood is thyrotoxicosis, which is responsible for clinical syndrome of hypermetabolism, sympathetic hyperactivity. Hyperthyroidism is the term used to denote the overproduction of thyroid hormones from the thyroid gland. Hyperthyroidism is possible with hyperactive thyroid gland due to multi/solitary nodular thyroid disease or Grave's disease. Thyrotoxicosis associated with thyroiditis is not hyperthyroidism. Treatment of hyperthyroidism is with anti-thyroid drugs (ATT), radio-active iodine ablation (RAI), or thyroid surgery; whereas, treatment of thyroiditis is symptomatic.

Keywords: thyrotoxicosis, hyperthyroidism, thyroiditis, anti-thyroid drugs (ATT), radio-active iodine ablation (RAI)

1. Introduction

Thyroid gland is a butterfly shaped gland located in front of neck. Thyroid gland synthesises and secretes thyroxine under influence of thyroid stimulating hormone (TSH). Hyperproduction and secretion of thyroxine is called as hyperthyroidism and presence of excess amount of thyroxine in blood is called as thyrotoxicosis. Hence presence of thyrotoxicosis does not necessarily means presence of hyperthyroidism, as thyrotoxicosis can be due to other reasons like thyroiditis, overdose of thyroxine tablets, ectopic sources like strauma ovarii producing excess thyroxine, etc. An approach to diagnose thyrotoxicosis is shown in **Figure 1**.

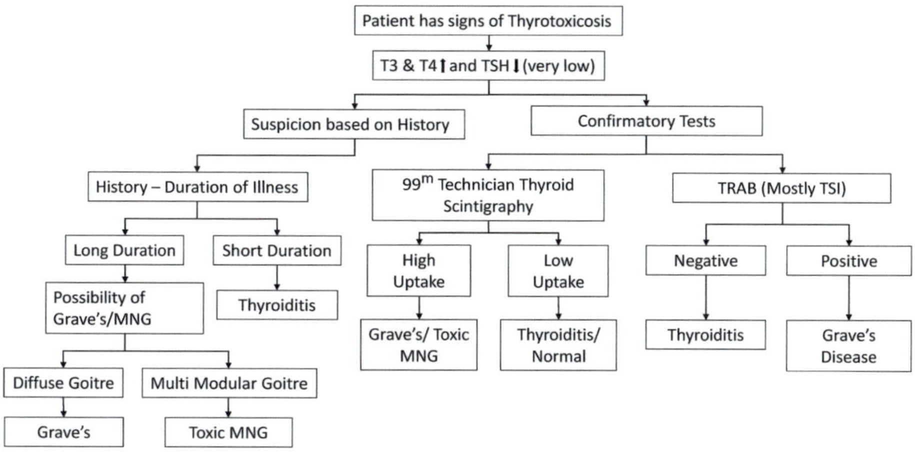

Figure 1.
Approach to thyrotoxicosis.

Treatment of thyrotoxicosis is symptomatic and the treatment of the cause, but treatment of hyperthyroidism is divided in three parts. First antithyroid drugs (ATD), radioactive iodine and thyroid surgery. The prevalence of hyperthyroidism is 1.2–1.6, 0.5–0.6 overt and 0.7–1.0% subclinical [1, 2]. The most frequent causes are Graves' disease (GD) and toxic nodular goitre.

1.1 Prevalence

Prevalence of thyroid disease varies with iodine sufficiency of the region The National health and nutrition examination survey (NHANES III) [3] and epidemic survey in UK [4] demonstrates female preponderance of thyroid diseases and lower incidence of hyperthyroidism with 1–2% prevalence in women and 1/10th in men.

2. Clinical manifestations

Hyperthyroidism can mimic other health problems, which can make it difficult to diagnose. It can also cause a wide variety of signs and symptoms like, Unintentional weight loss, palpitations, missed heartbeats, increased appetite, nervousness, anxiety and irritability, tremulousness, excess sweating, menstrual irregularity, heat intolerance, changes in bowel patterns especially more frequent bowel movements, goitre, easy fatigue, muscular weakness, insomnia, thinning of skin, hair loss. Elderly are either asymptomatic or may have palpitations, easy fatigue, etc.

Signs include tremors, warm handshake, fast tachycardia/arrhythmia, flushing over upper body, brisk reflexes, goitre and prominent eyes. Early diagnosis has become possible because of easy availability of blood investigations for thyroid.

Cause of patient's thyrotoxicosis can be guessed from presentation of patient and disease duration. Patients with hyperthyroidism have symptoms since months and dating back is usually difficult, patients of acute thyrotoxicosis due to thyroiditis usually date back their signs and symptoms. Many patients having mild thyrotoxicosis attribute their symptoms to day to day fatigue, stress, etc.

Easy access to blood tests of thyroid has made diagnosis of thyrotoxicosis easy. It is important to differentiate between thyrotoxicosis and hyperthyroidism before anti thyroid drugs are initiated.

Clinical manifestations involve multiple systems of the body as follows.

2.1 Cardiovascular system

Alterations in cardiovascular function are due to increased circulatory demand that result from the hyper metabolism, first, in heart rate, and with more severe disease, in stroke volume [5]. Widening of the pulse pressure results from the increase in systolic and decrease in diastolic pressure due to reduced peripheral resistance [6, 7].

2.2 Protein, carbohydrate, and lipid metabolism

Both synthesis and degradation rates of proteins are increased indicated by muscle wasting. Uncontrolled diabetes can be due to increased degradation rate of insulin. Lipolysis is predominantly observed [8].

2.3 Sympathetic nervous system and catecholamines

The improvement in cardiac function with β-blockade in patients with hyperthyroidism has led to the concept that there is increased sympathetic tone or increased cardiac sensitivity to the sympathetic nervous system in these patients [9].

2.4 Nervous system

Nervousness, emotional lability, and hyperkinesia are major symptoms.

Emotional lability mental disturbance may be severe; the patient shifts positions frequently, and movements are quick, jerky, exaggerated, and often purposeless.

In children, inability to focus may lead to deterioration of school performance. A fine tremor of the hands, tongue, or lightly closed eyelids is observed on clinical examination.

2.5 Muscle

Generalised wasting associated with weight loss. The weakness is most prominent in the proximal muscles of the limbs, myopathy is also a feature of disease which involves distal muscles, ocular myopathy may mimic myasthenia gravis. Periodic paralysis of the hypokalemic type may occur together with thyrotoxicosis [10–12].

2.6 Eyes

As shown in **Figure 2**, proptosis, stare, lid lag, globe lag, dry eyes, photosensitivity, corneal ulceration, loss of vision (uncommon) are features of Graves associated orbitopathy (GAO) [13].

2.7 Skin and hair

Excessive sweating. Palmar erythema may resemble "liver palms," and telangiectasia may be present. Hair loss may increase. The nails are often soft and friable. A characteristic but uncommon finding is Plummer's nails, or onycholysis, typically involving the fourth and fifth fingers [11].

2.8 Respiratory system

Dyspnoea is common in severe thyrotoxicosis, mainly from weakness of the respiratory muscles.

2.9 Alimentary system

An increase in appetite is common but is inadequate to meet the increased caloric requirements. The frequency of bowel movements is increased and hepatic dysfunction occurs [14]. Hepatomegaly and jaundice can develop with severe, prolonged disease, and liver failure was a cause of death before the development of successful treatment for patients with Graves' disease.

2.10 Haematopoietic system

The increase in erythropoiesis results from both a direct effect of thyroid hormones on the erythroid marrow and increased production of erythropoietin. Association of pernicious anaemia can be there in 3% of Graves of which 3% have auto-antibodies to intrinsic factor; accelerated clearance of the vitamin K-dependent clotting factors. Therefore, the dosage of warfarin needs to be reduced in thyotoxicosis [15].

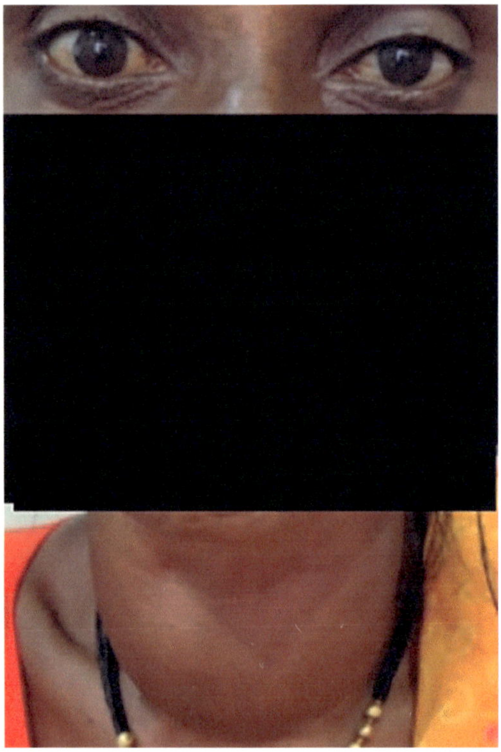

Figure 2.
Patient of Graves disease showing diffuse goitre and eye signs.

2.11 Reproductive function

Menstrual irregularity is common. Fertility may be reduced, and if conception takes place, there is an increased risk of miscarriage [16, 17]. The increased rate of conversion of androgens to estrogenic by-products may be the mechanism for gynecomastia and erectile dysfunction.

3. Graves' disease

Popularly known as Robert Graves' disease in English speaking world and as Von Basedow's disease in Europe, although disease was first described by Parry in 1825 [11].

3.1 Presentation

Graves' disease characteristics include goitre and thyrotoxicosis; common associated features include orbitopathy (GAO) and dermopathy. The thyroid histology suggests autoimmune thyroiditis with the presence of lymphocytic infiltrate.

4. Pathogenesis

4.1 The major antigen of Graves' disease: the thyrotropin receptor

The TSHR is a G protein coupled receptor. The TSHR is the primary auto antigen of Graves' disease, experimentally proven with mice antigen antibody studies [18].

5. Diagnosis

It is always better to test TSH and T4 rather than testing TSH alone, measuring both T4 & TSH increases diagnostic accuracy. In case of overt hyperthyroidism T3 and T4 are high and TSH is low and in subclinical disease T4 is usually normal TSH is usually suppressed, and T3 is normal or increased.

TSH-Receptor-Ab (TRAb) is a specific biomarker for Grave's Disease. Immunoassays used nowadays do competitive assays which measure Thyroid Receptor binding inhibitory immunoglobulins (TBII) [19]. Bioassays can differentiate between blocking and stimulating TRAB but its time consuming and a costly affair.

5.1 Imaging

Most clinicians would request thyroid ultrasound (US) and often isotope scanning is seldom available in India. Imaging tests are investigator dependant and hence experience and qualification of a person doing the test does matter, also matter is instruments used, hence a high-frequency linear probe should be used. GD is often, but not invariably, characterised by diffuse thyroid enlargement and by hypoechogenicity, both of which are assessed by ultra-sonogram and conventional grey scale analysis [20].

A colour-flow or power Doppler examination is characterised by vascular patterns and can quantify vascularity of thyroid [21]. Thyroid vascularity is significantly increased in severe Grave's disease and it typically shows a pulsatile pattern in thyroid gland which is called as "thyroid inferno" that is multiple small areas of increased intrathyroidal flow seen throughout the gland [22]. To measure accurately thyroid artery flow velocity and peak systolic velocity (PSV), it requires adjustments of pulse repetition frequency of wall filters and control of the insonation angle between 0 and 60°. The PSV is capable of differentiation between GD related thyrotoxicosis or amiodarone-induced thyrotoxicosis type 2, where the blood flow is reduced [23]. A typical US finding along with TRAB results can make diagnosis almost certain but thyroid scintigraphy is needed prior to Radioactive iodine ablation so that multinodular goitre can be differentiated [20].

6. Medical treatment

There are three ways by which GD is treated. One is by oral treatment with antithyroid drugs which reduces synthesis of thyroid hormones second is Radioactive iodine ablation where radioactive iodine is used to burn thyroid follicles and third one being thyroid surgery where thyroid gland is removed so that thyroid synthesising machinery is taken outside the body [20, 24]. ATD represent the most commonly used therapy in Europe, Asia, and in the meantime in the USA [25, 26]. The main ATD are thionamides, such as propylthiouracil (PTU), carbimazole (CBZ), and the active metabolite of the CBZ as, methimazole (MMI). CBZ is not an active substance; it has to be decarboxylated to MMI in the liver. Thionamides inhibit the coupling of iodothyronines and hence reduce the biosynthesis of TH [27]. These drugs mainly inhibit function of thyroperoxidase, reducing oxidation and the organification of iodide. ATD are indicated as a first-line treatment of GD, particularly in younger subjects, and for short-term treatment of GD before definitive RAI therapy or thyroidectomy [20]. ATD also helps to reduce TRAb levels and rates of remission of GD. PTU at very high doses also inhibits deiodination of T4 to T3 [28]. However, this effect is of use in case of thyrotoxicosis crisis but for long term use this effect is not of much use. The starting dose of MMI is usually 10–30 mg daily in divided doses depending on the severity of hyperthyroidism (CBZ 15–60 mg/day). PTU is given 100 mg every 8 h. titration regimen is used through the Corse of disease, means as disease goes in remission, dose is gradually reduced based on severity of the illness. Thyroid function tests are reviewed 3–4 weekly intervals after initial treatment, and the dose is titrated based on T4 and T3 levels. TSH values remain suppressed for long time hence more reliable is T3 & T4 reports but measuring T4 does add value to report as sometimes overtreatment increases TSH values in short span. The usual daily maintenance doses of ATD in the titration regimen are 2.5–10 mg of MMI and 50–100 mg of PTU. Some have also advocated block and replacement regimen to avoid severe hypothyroidism during treatment where MMZ in dose of 30–50 mg daily along with thyroxin replacement is used throughout the Corse but side effects of ATD are more with this kind of regimen [28].

6.1 Adverse events

Common side effects of ATD are allergic reactions which include rash, urticaria, and arthralgia (1–5%). Minor cutaneous reactions are managed with antihistaminics without stopping the ATD. Substituting an ATD may also be helpful [28]. In the case of a serious allergic reaction like hepatitis, a lupus-like syndrome, and agranulocytosis (neutrophil count <500/mL), which occurs in 0.1–1.0% of cases, it's better to avoid ATD in patients as risk of severity of allergic reaction may increase and it's better to use alternative ways of treatment [29]. Agranulocytosis may occur abruptly within 3 months after the initiation of ATD therapy [30]. The risk of ATD-induced agranulocytosis and pancytopenia at 100 and 150 days after the initiation of ATD was 0.28 and 0.29%, respectively [31].

6.2 Beta adrenergic drugs (β blockers)

These drugs are used as second line treatment of adjunctive treatment. These reduce catecholamine response at receptor level hence this is a symptomatic treatment and not a definitive treatment. Tremulousness, palpitations, excessive sweating, eyelid retraction, and heart rate decrease; by reducing sympathetic hyperactivity which is induces by excess TH in blood. Propranolol (but not other β-adrenergic agents) may also weakly block the conversion of T4 to T3 via a mechanism independent of its effect on catecholamine signalling. Propranolol is the most widely used agent because it is relatively free from adverse effects and has a short half-life. It can be given orally in a dose of 20–60 mg every 6 or 8 h and avoided in patients with known history of bronchial asthma or COPD with respiratory problems. Hypotension with Propranolol is unusual [32].

6.3 Radioablation

Introduced in the mid-1940s, a relatively inexpensive therapy for treatment of hyperthyroidism, 131I has become the most widely used therapy, although international questionnaire studies show that geographic differences do exist. The isotope being used is 131I. It is given orally (in a capsule or in water) and is absorbed rapidly and completely, after which it is concentrated, oxidised, and organified by follicular thyroid cells. The ionising effect of β-particles, with a path length of 1–2 mm, destroys the thyroid cells by an early inflammatory response, necrosis of follicular cells, and vascular occlusion. Further chronic inflammation and fibrosis result in a decrease in thyroid size and an impaired thyroid function. So most of the patients developed Hypothyroidism following 131I therapy [33].

6.4 Dose calculation

Smallest possible dose is preferred so that to make patients euthyroid and avoid permanent hypothyroidism in patients. Dose is calculated by following algorithm:

Dose (mCi) = (80 - 200 micro Ci 131I/g thyroid × estimated thyroid gland weight (g) ÷ 24 h radioiodine uptake).

With use of above dose calculation algorithm, usual dose patients receive is 5–15 mCi and many become euthyroid followed by hypothyroidism. Dose calculation is time consuming and costly hence fixed dose activity is commonly used in many centres which simplifies and reduces cost of 131I therapy and the lack of a significant difference in outcome between patients randomised to fixed and calculated 131I doses favour the use of fixed doses. Typically a patient with Graves' disease requires 5–15 mCi, 10–29 mCi in patients with toxic nodule and toxic MNG [33]. Not all patients respond to 131I and these patients may require multiple doses at 6–12 monthly intervals. Patients who can be predicted to have poor response are: (1) age (>40 years); (2) Gender (female); (3) severe hyperthyroidism; (4) medium or large goitres (>40 g, visible); and (5) ATD pre-treatment (especially with propylthiouracil) [34].

6.5 Surgery

Thyroid surgery is oldest available treatment for hyperthyroidism and it's a definitive treatment for the illness. Being an invasive treatment and also associated complications, its least preferred now a days, but indications for the treatment include: (1) patients preference; (2) large size goitres which are causing compressive symptoms or for cosmetic reasons; (3) Graves' disease super imposed on endemic goitre with multiple cold nodules; (4) suspicion of malignancy; and (5) associated with ophthalmopathy.

6.6 Pre-operative preparation

It is mandatory to achieve normal metabolic state before patients undergo thyroid surgery or else patients may land u into thyroid storm. Normal metabolic state is generally achieved by using ATD in appropriate dose and duration. Beta blockers are also used in management to achieve eumetabolism before surgery. Once eumetabolism is achieved SSKI is added, 2–3 drops twice daily, for 7–10 days. Lugol's iodine can also be used depending on its availability.

6.7 Treatment of sub-acute thyroiditis

Treatment is usually supportive and symptomatic. Pain is relieved with NSAID's. If pain persists despite maximal NSAID's, prednisolone in a dose of 40 mg per day for 7–10 days is followed [35].

7. Special situation

7.1 Hyperthyroidism in pregnancy

Hyperthyroidism is not uncommon during pregnancy with prevalence being 0.1–0.4% of which 80% of the cases are of Grave's disease. The activity level of Graves' disease fluctuate during gestation, with exacerbation during the first trimester and improvement by late gestation related to autoimmune process of the disease affected by gestation. Hyperthyroidism of Graves' disease may also be aggravated by high levels of HCG in the first trimester. Because nonspecific symptoms of hyperthyroidism may be mimicked by normal pregnancy, the presence of a goitre, especially with a bruit or thrill, which may point to a diagnosis of true Graves' disease. One has to be cautious before labelling diagnosis of Grave's disease and should first rule out gestational thyrotoxicosis [36–38].

Patients suspected of having hyperthyroidism require measurement of serum TSH, T4, T3 levels, and TRAb. And it's always necessary to interpret thyroid function tests in relation to the HCG-mediated decrease in serum TSH levels and the increase in T4 binding globulin concentrations that occur during normal pregnancy [39–41].

In a normal pregnancy TSH is typically suppressed specially during late first trimester and last trimester, a lady with Graves' disease, one must anticipate transplacental transfer of TRAB and fetal hyperthyroidism hence adequate treatment of a pregnant woman is necessary to avoid fetal hyperthyroidism. Fetal hyperthyroidism and inadequate treatment is associated with increased risk of medically indicated preterm delivery, intrauterine growth restriction and low birth weight, pre-eclampsia, congestive heart failure, and fetal death [42]. In addition, overtreatment of the mother with thionamides can result in iatrogenic fetal hypothyroidism [43], but under treatment of maternal hyperthyroidism may lead to central congenital hypothyroidism [44, 45].

Fetal hyperthyroidism is known to be associated with intrauterine growth restriction, fetal tachycardia, fetal goitre, advanced bone age, fetal hydrops, preterm delivery, and fetal death [46]. The diagnosis is suggested by any of these signs or abnormalities. Maternal TRAb levels able to induce fetal hyperthyroidism are usually over three times the upper normal limit. PTU and MMI or its derivative carbimazole are the mainstays of treatment. Recently, the Adverse Event Reporting System of the FDA has focused attention on the relation between hepatotoxicity and PTU [47]. This finding has led to a recommendation that PTU use in pregnancy should be limited to the first trimester, and then treatment must be switched to MMI. Use of MMI during the first trimester has been associated with a possible embryopathy.

Author details

Rushikesh Maheshwari
Private Practice at Rushikesh Endocare Superspeciality Centre, Nanded, Maharashtra, India

*Address all correspondence to: rushikeshmaheshwari@gmail.com

References

[1] Bahn RS, Burch HB, Cooper DS, et al. Management guidelines of the American Thyroid Association and American Association of Clinical Endocrinologists. Endocrine Practice. 2011;**17**:456-520

[2] Ross DS, Burch HB, Cooper DS, Greenlee MC, Laurberg P, et al. 2016 American Thyroid Association guidelines for diagnosis and management of hyperthyroidism and other causes of thyrotoxicosis. Thyroid. 2016;**26**:1343-1421

[3] Vanderpump NPJ et al. The incidence of thyroid disorder in community: A twenty year follow up of Whikham survey. Clinical Endocrinology. 1995;**43**:55-68

[4] Carlae A, Pederson IB, et al. Epidemiology of subtypes of hyperthyroidism in Denmark, a population based study. European Journal of Endocrinology. 2011;**164**:801-809

[5] Burggraaf J, Tulen JH, Lalezari S, et al. Sympathovagal imbalance in hyperthyroidism. American Journal of Physiology. Endocrinology and Metabolism. 2001;**281**:E190-E195

[6] Fazio S, Palmieri EA, Lombardi G, et al. Effects of thyroid hormone on the cardiovascular system. Recent Progress in Hormone Research. 2004;**59**:31-50

[7] Kahaly GJ, Wagner S, Nieswandt J, et al. Stress echocardiography in hyperthyroidism. The Journal of Clinical Endocrinology and Metabolism. 1999;**84**:2308-2313

[8] Silva JE. The thermogenic effect of thyroid hormone and its clinical implications. Annals of Internal Medicine. 2003;**139**:205-213

[9] Keating FR, Parkin TW, Selby JB, et al. Treatment of heart disease associated with myxedema. Progress in Cardiovascular Diseases. 1961;**3**:364-381

[10] Imaizumi M, Akahoshi M, Ichimaru S, et al. Risk for ischemic heart disease and all-cause mortality in subclinical hypothyroidism. The Journal of Clinical Endocrinology and Metabolism. 2004;**89**:3365-3370

[11] Cappola AR, Fried LP, Arnold AM, et al. Thyroid status, cardiovascular risk, and mortality in older adults. Journal of the American Medical Association. 2006;**295**:1033-1041

[12] Tachman ML, Guthrie GP Jr. Hypothyroidism: Diversity of presentation. Endocrine Reviews. 1984;**5**:456-465

[13] Mandel SJ, Larsen PR, Davies TF. Thyrotoxicosis. In: Williams Textbook of Endocrinology. 12th ed. Philadelphia, PA: Elsevier Saunders. pp. 366-400

[14] Checchi S, Montanaro A, Pasqui L, et al. L-Thyroxine requirement in patients with auotimmune hypothyroidism and parietal cell antibodies. The Journal of Clinical Endocrinology and Metabolism. 2008;**93**:465-469

[15] Lecky BRF, Williams TDM, Lightman SL, et al. Myxoedema presenting with chiasmal compression: Resolution after thyroxine replacement. Lancet. 1987;**1**:1347-1350

[16] Redmond GP. Thyroid dysfunction and women's reproductive health. Thyroid. 2004;**14**(Suppl):S5-S15

[17] Yoshimura M, Hershman JM. Thyrotropic action of human chorionic gonadotropin. Thyroid. 1995;**5**:425-434

[18] Shimojo N, Kohno Y, et al. Induction of Graves like disease in mice by immunization with fibroblasts

transfected with the thyrotropin receptor and a class II molecule. Proceedings of the National Academy of Sciences of the United States of America. 1996;**93**:11074-11079

[19] Bartalena L. Diagnosis and management of Grave's disease: A global overview. Nature Reviews. Endocrinology. 2013;**9**:724-734

[20] Smith TJ, Hegedus L. Graves' disease. The New England Journal of Medicine. 2016;**375**:1552-1565

[21] Erdogan MF, Anil C, et al. Colour flow Doppler sonography for the etiologic diagnosis of hyperthyroidism. Thyroid. 2007;**17**:223-228

[22] Ralls PW et al. Color-flow Doppler sonography in Grave's disease. American Journal of Roentgenology. 1988;**150**:781-784

[23] Kim TK, Lee EJ. The value of the mean peak systolic velocity of the superior thyroidal artery in the differential diagnosis of thyrotoxicosis. Ultrasonography. 2015;**34**:292-296

[24] Kahaly GJ, Bartalena L, Hegedus L. The American Thyroid Association/American Association of Clinical Endocrinologists guidelines for hyperthyroidism and other causes of thyrotoxicosis: A European perspective. Thyroid. 2011;**21**:585-591

[25] Emiliano AB, Governale L, et al. Shifts in PTU and MMI prescribing practices. JCEM. 2010;**95**:2227-2233

[26] Brito JP et al. Antithyroid drugs—The most common treatment for Graves' disease in the US: A nationwide population-based study. Thyroid. 2016;**26**:1144-1145

[27] Cooper DS. Antithyroid drugs in the management of patients with Graves' disease. JCEM. 2003;**88**:3474-3481

[28] Cooper DS. Antithyroid drugs. NEJM. 2005;**352**:905-917

[29] Pearce SH. Spontaneous reporting of adverse reactions to carbimazole and propylthiouracil in the UK. Clinical Endocrinology. 2004;**61**:589-594

[30] Nakamura H, Miyauchi A, et al. Analysis of 754 cases of antithyroid drug-induced agranulocytosis over 30 years in Japan. JCEM. 2013;**98**:4776-4783

[31] Watanabe N et al. Antithyroid drug induced hematopoietic damage. JCEM. 2012;**97**:E49-E53

[32] Geffner DL, Hershman JM. Beta-adrenergic blockade for the treatment of hyperthyroidism. The American Journal of Medicine. 1992;**93**(1):61-68

[33] Suryanarayana KM. Hyperthyroidism: Relevant investigations and guidelines for management. Medicine Update. 2010;**20**:440-445

[34] Allahabadia A, Daykin J, Sheppard MC, et al. Radioiodine treatment of hyperthyroidism—Prognostic factors for outcome. The Journal of Clinical Endocrinology and Metabolism. 2001;**86**(8):3611-3617

[35] Elizabeth PN, Alan FP, Lewis BE. Thyroiditis. The New England Journal of Medicine. 2003;**348**:2646-2655

[36] Mandel SJ, Cooper DS. The use of antithyroid drugs in pregnancy and lactation. The Journal of Clinical Endocrinology and Metabolism. 2001;**86**:2354-2359

[37] Glinoer D. Thyroid hyperfunction during pregnancy. Thyroid. 1998; **8**:859-864

[38] Niswander KR, Gordon M, editors. The Collaborative Perinatal Study of the National Institute of Neurologic Disease

and Stroke. Philadelphia: WB Saunders; 1972. pp. 246-249

[39] de Glinoer D et al. Regulation of maternal thyroid during pregnancy. JCEM. 1990;**71**:276-287

[40] Glinoer D, De Nayer P, Robyn C, Lejeune B, Kinthaert J, Meuris S. Serum levels of intact human chorionic gonadotropin (HCG) and its free and subunits, in relation to maternal thyroid stimulation during normal pregnancy. Journal of Endocrinological Investigation. 1993;**16**:881-888

[41] Hershman JM. Human chorionic gonadotropin and the thyroid: Hyperemesis gravidarum and trophoblastic tumors. Thyroid. 1999;**9**:653-657

[42] Millar LK, Wing DA, Leung AS, Koonings PP, Montoro MN, Mestman JH. Low birth weight and preeclampsia in pregnancies complicated by hyperthyroidism. Obstetrics and Gynecology. 1994;**84**:946-949

[43] Davidson KM, Richards DS, Schatz DA, Fisher DA. Successful in utero treatment of fetal goiter and hypothyroidism. The New England Journal of Medicine. 1991;**324**:543-546

[44] Kempers MJ, van Tijn DA, van Trotsenburg AS, de Vijlder JJ, Wiedijk BM, Vulsma T. Central congenital hypothyroidism due to gestational hyperthyroidism: Detection where prevention failed. The Journal of Clinical Endocrinology and Metabolism. 2003;**88**:5851-5857

[45] Papendieck P, Chiesa A, Prieto L, Gruñeiro-Papendieck L. Thyroid disorders of neonates born to mothers with Graves' disease. Journal of Pediatric Endocrinology & Metabolism. 2009;**22**:547-553

[46] De Groot L, Abalovich M, Erik K, et al. Management of thyroid dysfunction during pregnancy and postpartum: An Endocrine Society Clinical Practice guideline. The Journal of Clinical Endocrinology and Metabolism. 2012;**97**:2543-2565

[47] Cooper DS, Rivkees SA. Putting propylthiouracil in perspective. The Journal of Clinical Endocrinology and Metabolism. 2009;**94**:1881-1882

Chapter 5

Prevention and Treatment of Iodine-Induced Thyrotoxicosis

Melinda Kolcsár and Zsolt Gáll

Abstract

Etiologies of thyrotoxicosis are diverse, one of them being caused by iodine-induced hyperthyroidism. The clinical signs of the disease are the classical signs of any form of hyperthyroidism, but the treatment of the different forms presents particular aspects. This chapter reviews the risk factors for thyrotoxicosis following an excess iodine load, pointing out the major sources of iodine: supplementation programs, dietary intake, nutritional supplements, iodine-containing contrast medium, and amiodarone. Prevention of iodine-induced thyrotoxicosis is critical in geriatric patients who often have thyroid nodular disease, underlying heart conditions, and therefore, hyperthyroidism may be more difficult to detect clinically. Treatment of iodine-induced thyrotoxicosis could be performed with thioamides or perchlorate prior to the administration of an iodine containing product (e.g., food, dietary supplements, and contrast media). On the other hand, amiodarone-induced thyrotoxicosis needs further attention and a close collaboration between cardiology and endocrinology to overcome complications, but individualization of the therapy should be undertaken. Based on the specific features of amiodarone-induced thyrotoxicosis thioamides, perchlorate, high-dose glucocorticoids, or radioiodine therapy may be considered for an optimal therapeutic intervention.

Keywords: iodine deficiency, iodine supplementation, dietary iodine, iodine containing contrast media, amiodarone, thyrotoxicosis, thioamides, perchlorate, glucocorticoids

1. Introduction

Thyroxine (T4) and 3,5,3′-triiodothyronine (T3) are the two thyroid hormones, each of them containing two iodine atoms on their inner (tyrosine) ring. The difference between them is that T3 has only one iodine atom on its outer (phenyl) ring, whereas T4 has two. Synthesis of reasonable quantities of thyroid hormones requires adequate iodine intake to allow sufficient thyroidal uptake. The World Health Organization (WHO) recommendation for daily intake of iodine is 90 μg for infants and children up to 5 years, 120 μg for children 6–12 years, 150 μg for children ≥12 years and adults, and 250 μg for pregnant and lactating women [1]. The worldwide variability of the dietary intake of iodine depends on the iodine content of the soil, water, and the dietary practice. After Iodine Global Network data [2], the iodine uptake in Romania in 2004 was considered adequate, the median urinary iodine content (MUIC, normal value ≥100 μg/L) being 102 μg/L in school-aged children, but in some geographic regions, such as mountainous villages of Mureș County, a mild iodine deficiency was detected [3]. The MUIC value (68 μg/L) in pregnant women confirmed that iodine intake in this population of Romania is insufficient [2]. Administration of supplemental iodine to subjects with iodine deficiency goiter can result in iodine-induced hyperthyroidism in nonpregnant persons [4], but iodine supplementation in mild and moderate iodine-deficient pregnant women lowers thyroid hormone level [5].

2. Risk factors for thyrotoxicosis following an iodine load

2.1 Normal adaptation to iodine intake

Thyroid hormone secretion is regulated by two mechanisms: a central hypothalamic-pituitary and a local autoregulatory mechanism depending on the iodine content of the gland. The autoregulatory mechanism reduces the fluctuation of thyroid hormone secretion in the event of sudden changes in iodine supply. Iodine excess inhibits iodide accumulation, organogenesis, tyrosine binding, and thyroid hormone release. However, this inhibitory effect (Wolff-Chaikoff effect) lasts only 10–14 days, followed by the so-called escape phenomenon [6].

Iodine is a micronutrient that is present in foods (e.g., seaweed, seafood, dairy- and grain products, eggs), added to processed foods as iodized salt, and available as a dietary supplement, but the iodine concentration of water and foods is highly variable. Studies of iodine balance, based on the assumption that a healthy subject on an adequate diet maintains equilibrium between iodine intake and losses, have provided highly variable results, thus, cannot be used for setting daily reference values [7]. When iodine losses exceed intake (negative balance), deposits are progressively depleted resulting in biological signs and in clinical symptoms of deficiency. The physiological response to iodine deficiency is the preferential synthesis of T3 instead of T4. Long-term follow-up suggests that chronic iodine deficiency may lead to insufficient thyroid function (hypothyroidism) associated with a compensatory thyroid hypertrophy/hyperplasia with goiter (enlarged thyroid gland). Myxedema, observed with severe iodine deficiency, also results from hormone deficiency and is associated with reduced metabolic rate, weight gain, swollen face, edemas, hypothermia, and mental slowness. In euthyroid subjects, the plasma concentration of iodine (inorganic and organic iodine) ranged from 40 to 80 μg/L. Concentrations between 80 and 250 μg/L are associated with hyperthyroidism, whereas concentrations above 250 μg/L usually result from iodine overload with iodinated drugs [8, 9]. The thyroid gland, being highly flexible, is able to concentrate iodine up to 80-fold, and in most healthy adults, no clinical signs will appear at an iodine intake of up to 2 g/day [10]. However, if the adaptation to high iodine intake fails, various diseases occur. Chronic excessive iodine supply can also lead to goiter [11] and may accelerate the development of subclinical thyroid disorders to overt hypothyroidism or hyperthyroidism, increase the incidence of autoimmune thyroiditis, and increase the risk of thyroid cancer [10, 12, 13]. Recently, high iodine intake (exceeding 160 μg daily) was suggested as a risk factor for type 2 diabetes [14].

2.2 Iodine-induced thyrotoxicosis mechanisms

Iodine-induced hyperthyroidism (thyrotoxicosis) or Jod-Basedow effect is most frequently observed following iodine supplementation in individuals who had previously experienced severe iodine deficiency [15, 16]. A plausible explanation of this phenomenon can be the thyroid stimulating hormone (TSH) hyperstimulation of the thyroid gland, which may occur as an adaptive response to the iodine-deficient conditions and results in autonomous growth and function of thyrocyte clusters. When iodine intake increases, these nodules may synthesize an excessive amount of thyroid hormones [10]. The mechanism consists of escape phenomenon when high doses of iodine are used for thyroid hormone synthesis, which can lead to severe thyrotoxicosis. The high iodine containing amiodarone and its metabolite N-desethylamiodarone (DEA) affects T cell function by increasing the number of both helper and cytotoxic T lymphocytes and induces destructive thyroiditis, resulting in transient thyrotoxicosis, as suggested by clinical, histological, and in vitro studies [17–19].

High levels of organic iodide (thyroid hormones) also reduce the accumulation of iodide ions in the thyroid gland inhibiting the TSH secretion.

The effects of iodine administration differ in patients with pre-existing thyroid pathology from those in healthy subjects and depend upon the underlying disease process.

3. Major sources of increased iodine exposure: iodine supplementation, dietary iodine, iodine-containing contrast media, amiodarone, and the clinical forms of amiodarone-induced thyrotoxicosis

3.1 Iodine supplementation

The assessment of iodine deficiency can be accomplished by assessing the prevalence and severity of goiter, by testing the excretion of iodine in urine, and by determining hormonal levels (e.g., TSH, FT4). When used alone, neither of these are sufficiently sensitive and specific to measure iodine deficiency of a population, but urinary iodine remains the index of choice in the monitoring of iodine supplementation programmes. The most successful method of intervention for iodine deficiency control is salt iodization, iodine being added to salt as potassium iodide (KI), potassium iodate (KIO_3), or sodium iodide (NaI). Due to the high prevalence of hypertension and cardiovascular diseases, many countries proposed to promote the reduction of salt intake to 5 g/day (<2 g of sodium), so complementary measures are needed in order to tackle iodine deficiency [20]. But iodine also binds to fatty acids, so iodine oil can also be given orally or intravenously to severely iodine-deficient patients in the short term. Nascent iodine is like the precursor form of iodine, which converts into thyroid hormones. The human body can recognize and assimilate this form more easily than potassium salt. Lugol's solution is a widely used commercial iodine source, which contains elemental iodine and potassium iodide also. If someone consumes high quantities of iodine-rich foods (e.g., marine food, kelp), the use of iodized salt or iodinated water may increase iodine levels above the safe upper level as recommended by WHO. Individuals, who consume large amounts of seaweed regularly, are also exposed to the risk of iodine-induced hyperthyroidism [21, 22]. Several reports are available describing diet-induced thyrotoxicosis in patients consuming seaweed-containing foods or beverages [23]. Risk factors for iodineinduced hyperthyroidism include nontoxic or diffuse nodular goiter, latent Graves' disease, and long-standing iodine deficiency [24].

3.2 Dietary supplements

Most dietary supplements, as well as food and water, contains iodine as salts: sodium iodide, sodium iodate, potassium iodide, and potassium iodate. Different solid dosage forms of potassium iodide are available, but around 20% is assimilated from inorganic forms of iodine into the body [25]. Iodine is also present in most multivitamin/mineral supplements. Some case reports described that previously

Nutritional supplement	Iodine content per serving (µg)	% RDA iodine per serving (%)
Natural Living Iodine Plus-2®	12500	8333
Terry Naturally® (Europharma) Tri-Iodine®	25000, 12500, 6250, 3000	16667, 8333, 4167, 2000
Oradix StemDetox™	5000	3333
Survival shield X-2, Detoxadine® (nascent iodine)	1950	1300
Dr. Mercola Iodine	1500, 500	1000, 333
Life Extension® sea iodine	1000	667

Table 1.
Commercially available nutritional supplements with iodine content exceeding the daily intake recommended by WHO (RDA—recommended daily allowances).

euthyroid patients taking nutritional supplements developed iodine-induced hyperthyroidism [26–28]. The iodine content of dietary supplements shows high variability; some supplements may contain up to 160-fold of the recommended daily intake (**Table 1**). Short-term increase of basal and poststimulation TSH was described even in euthyroid patients administering dietary supplements with kelp [29, 30].

3.3 Iodine-containing contrast media

Iodinated contrast media (ICM) is given for computed tomography (CT), angiography, myelography, and arthrogram. The route of administration could be systemic as i.v, i.a., oral, rectal, and local. The pharmacokinetics of all currently available ICMs is similar. The half-life of ICM in normal renal function subjects is approximately 2 hours. Thus, approximately 20 hours are required for the total excretion of the administered ICM [31]. Referring to their iodine content and osmolarity, the contrast media are divided into ionic ICM with high osmolarity (1500–2000 mOsm/kg) or nonionic ICM with low and iso-osmolarity (600–1000 mOsm/kg). A list of iodinated contrast agents available in Romania and their molecular properties can be found in **Table 2**.

The safety profile of the systemic administered nonionic low- or iso-osmolar contrast currently in use is 5- to 10-fold better than the ionic high-osmolar agents [32, 33]. The ratio of iodine atoms to the number of contrast particles in low-osmolar solution is higher than compared with high osmolar ICM and hence have a greater concentration of iodine than the high osmolar [32]. In both low and high osmolar ICM, the iodine content is far greater than the recommended daily allowance. Patients generally are given 50 and 100 mL of contrast per CT scan; however, it is essential to know that not all CT scans require contrast media administration (see **Table 3**) [31, 33–35].

Higher doses of ICM may be required for invasive procedures such as cardiac catheterization. Typical doses for CT scans provide 2500–5000 µg of bioavailable free iodine and 15–37 g of total iodine [36]. Nonbioavailable iodine may be liberated to free iodide, particularly with increased half-times in the body (i.e., impaired kidney function) [35, 36]. After ICM administration, iodine deposits remain elevated for up to 4–8 weeks in patients with healthy thyroid. The urinary iodine excretion increased by 300–400% from baseline to peak levels after 1.1 week and normalized by 5.2 weeks following ICM administration [37].

After exposure to the iodine-containing contrast agent, the most rapid (hours to days) effect of pharmacologic doses of iodine is the Wolff-Chaikoff effect. The

Nonionic ICM	Iodine content, mg/mL	Osmolarity
Watersoluble, nephrotropic X-ray contrast media		
Iobitridol	300, 350	Low
Iodixanol	270, 320	Low
Iohexol	240, 300, 350	Low
Iomeprol	300, 350, 400	Low
Iopamidol	300, 370	Low
Iopromide	300, 370	Low
Ioversol	240, 300, 320, 350	Low
Non-watersoluble		
Ethiodized oil	480	

Table 2.
The iodine content of nonionic iodinated contrast media (ICM) and their molecular properties.

CT type	Contrast indicated	Contrast not indicated
Head	Neoplasm, meningitis, encephalitis, focal neurologic deficits, skull base disorders, orbital and vision disorders, pituitary imaging, complicated sinonasal disease, seizures, cerebral angiography	Head trauma, acute stroke, intracranial hemorrhage
Cervical	Cervical mass or lymphadenopathy, suspected tumor or infection, abnormalities of cranial nerves X, XI, and XII, brachial plexopathy	Trauma unless arterial injury is a possibility or the mechanism of injury is penetrating
Cardiothoracic	Heart and thoracic vessels, trauma, staging primary thoracic neoplasms	Coronary calcium scoring, pulmonary parenchymal evaluation lymph node evaluation
Abdominopelvic	Virtually all other gastrointestinal, hepatopancreaticobiliary, genitourinary, gynecologic indications	Colonography, renal stone evaluation, extraparenchymal lymphoma
Musculoskeletal	Evaluation of soft tissue masses and suspected septic arthritis or infected prostheses	Extremities and spine
CT angiography	Evaluating the lumen of an artery, vein, or a pseudoaneurysm and to assess for end-organ ischemia outside the brain or lung to detect active bleeding	Monitoring a known aneurysm for growth or for detection of a hematoma

Table 3.
Indications of contrast enhancement in CT imaging.

mechanism for this acute effect is partially explained by the generation of iodolactones, iodoaldehydes, and/or iodolipids, which inhibit thyroid peroxidase activity, necessary for thyroid hormone synthesis [37]. The decrease of thyroglobulin proteolysis resulting in reduced thyroid hormone secretion also may be contributing to the ICM-induced Wolff-Chaikoff effect. The diminished serum T4 and T3 concentrations temporarily increased the serum concentrations of TSH, in some cases above the normal range. The phenomenon is transient in euthyroid adult patients and does not typically determine permanent hypothyroidism [38].

ICM use could lead to thyroid dysfunction, namely to hypo- and hyperthyroidism. Iodine excess-induced hypothyroidism appears when the thyroid fails to escape from the acute Wolff-Chaikoff effect. It occurs in patients with a wide variety of underlying thyroid abnormalities, including Hashimoto's thyroiditis, previously treated Graves' disease, history of thyroid lobectomy, postpartum lymphocytic thyroiditis, interferon therapy, or type 2 amiodarone-induced thyrotoxicosis [12, 39, 40]. Not only the previous thyroid disorder but also the age of the patients is a contributing factor in hypothyroidism development. A systematic review evidenced that hospitalized neonates, especially premature infants exposed to iodinated contrast media, are at increased risk for development of hypothyroidism [41]. It could be hypothesized that hypothyroidism in this case to be partially secondary to an immature thyroid gland and an exaggerated Wolff-Chaikoff effect. Older age patients are also at high risk of developing hypothyroidism after ICM exposure, as reported in a study including the Asian population [42].

Patients with one exposure to ICM showed the highest risk of thyroid dysfunction compared with non-ICM exposure and a correlation was still found between the frequency of ICM exposure and the risk of hypothyroidism [42]. Conflicting data appear regarding to the time of onset of hypothyroidism after ICM administration: Rhee et al. [43] showed that the median time interval until the occurrence of hypothyroidism was 1 year, but Kornelius et al. [42] reported that hypothyroidism may develop 2.1 years after ICM exposure.

ICM-induced hyperthyroidism rarely occurs in individuals without prior thyroid dysfunction. Previously existent thyroid diseases, such as nodular goiter, Graves' disease, and long-standing iodine deficiency followed by thyroid autonomy, were reported to be associated with a higher risk of hyperthyroidism after ICM exposure [4, 13, 24, 36, 42]. The mechanism of ICM-induced hyperthyroidism involves impairment of the acute Wolff-Chaikoff effect due to rapid iodine excess and influx into the thyroid gland. Excess iodine intake will result in transient or permanent hyperthyroidism [13, 24, 42]. Kornelius et al. [42] found in their study a 22% increased risk of hyperthyroidism after ICM administration. Older patients (between 20 and 60 years) presented a more than twofold increased risk of hyperthyroidism compared with younger patients (less than 20 years old). The number of ICM exposures did not increase the risk of hyperthyroidism. It could be hypothesized that the "stunning effect" plays a certain role in hyperthyroidism, involving a diminished absorption of excess iodine in patients with repeated iodine exposure.

3.4 Amiodarone

3.4.1 Amiodarone pharmacology

Amiodarone is a class III antiarrhythmic agent, having short- and long-term actions on multiple molecular levels [44]. Its molecular structure resembles T3. However, amiodarone can alter thyroid function (inducing both hypo- and hyperthyroidism), which is due to amiodarone's high iodine content and its direct toxic effect on the thyroid follicle cells. Amiodarone is a benzofuran derivative with great lipophilicity, which is extensively distributed in adipose tissue, cardiac and skeletal muscle, liver, lung, and the thyroid. During its liver metabolization, approximately 6 mg of inorganic iodine per 200 mg of amiodarone ingested is released into the systemic circulation [45]. The average iodine content in Romanian diet is approximately 50–75 μg/day [3, 46, 47]. Thus, 6 mg of iodine markedly increases the daily iodine load. Amiodarone elimination from the body occurs with a half-life of approximately 55–100 days. The long half-life of both amiodarone and his active metabolite, DEA, contributes to his toxicity. For a therapeutic effect, a plasma concentration between 0.5 and 2.5 μg/mL is required; however, serum levels do not correlate well with efficacy or with adverse effects [45, 48–50].

3.4.2 Amiodarone and the thyroid

The effects of amiodarone on thyroid function can be divided into those effects that are due to iodine and those effects that are intrinsic properties of the drug.

3.4.2.1 Effects due to iodine

After chronic amiodarone administration, the thyroid dysfunctions may occur in 5–22% of the patients. Risk factors for the development of thyroid disease include not only treatment duration and cumulative amiodarone dose but also age, gender, pre-existing thyroid pathology, and associated nonthyroid conditions [51–53]. The normal autoregulation process of thyroid prevents normal individuals from becoming hyperthyroid after exposure to the high iodine content substances. When intrathyroidal iodine concentrations reach a critically high level, iodine transport and thyroid hormone synthesis are transiently inhibited until intrathyroidal iodine stores return to physiological levels (see the Wolff-Chaikoff effect). Patients with underlying thyroid pathology, however, have defects in autoregulation of iodine: for example, in autoimmune thyroid disease exists a "fail to escape" from the Wolff-Chaikoff effect. The result is the development of goiter and hypothyroidism in Hashimoto's disease. Patients with areas of autonomous function within a nodular goiter do not autoregulate iodine and the addition of more substrate may result in excessive thyroid hormone synthesis and thyrotoxicosis (see Iod-Basedow) [13, 54, 55].

3.4.2.2 Intrinsic drug effects

Amiodarone inhibits peripheral deiodinase (outer ring 5′-monodeiodination of T4), thus decreasing T3 production and increasing T4 level; reverse T3 (rT3) accumulates since it is not metabolized to T2 [4, 56, 57]; amiodarone and, particularly, the metabolite DEA block T3-receptor binding to nuclear receptors [58] and decrease the expression of some thyroid hormone-related genes [59]; amiodarone may have a direct cytotoxic effect on thyroid follicular structures, which results in a destructive thyroiditis [60]. Martino et al. described marked distortion of thyroid follicle architecture, necrosis, apoptosis, inclusion bodies, lipofuscinogenesis, markedly dilated endoplasmic reticulum, and macrophage infiltration after amiodarone [19]. The role of the pre-existing autoimmune process is widely debated, due to the conflicting results of the retrospective study data [17, 18, 55]. Even if amiodarone does not induce de novo autoimmune thyroid disease, by the direct cytotoxic effect, it may cause the release of pre-existing autoantibodies and thus worsen destructive thyroiditis. In a study [61], it was described that in women the prolonged amiodarone treatment (for over 2 years) increased the antithyroid peroxidase titer.

3.4.3 Risk of thyrotoxicosis after amiodarone administration

Predisposing factors for amiodarone-induced thyrotoxicosis include environmental factors such as dietary iodine (deficiency), as well as intrinsic factors such as pre-existing thyroid pathology. Depending on these factors, a great variability exists regarding the incidence of amiodarone-induced thyroid dysfunction ranges (5–22%) [51, 52, 62, 63].

Dietary iodine intake affects an individual's risk of amiodarone-induced thyroid dysfunction: in iodine-deficient areas, amiodarone-induced thyrotoxicosis (AIT) appears to be more common than hypothyroidism [64], whereas in iodine-sufficient areas, amiodarone-induced hypothyroidism is more common than hyperthyroidism [19]. The incidence of reported AIT in different studies varies but remains within the range of 5–10% in most studies [51, 52, 63]. As was reported in a previous study from the UK, AIT appears more frequently in men than in women [65], but the time of onset of AIT is unpredictable. It can occur at almost any time throughout the course of amiodarone treatment and last for as long as 6–9 months after treatment withdrawal, almost certainly because of the drug's long half-life and associated iodine load [66]. One study illustrates the importance of the underlying thyroid status near the dietary iodine intake in relation to the risk of developing amiodarone-induced thyroid dysfunction. In Worcester, Massachusetts, an area with iodine sufficiency and a high prevalence of autoimmune thyroid disease, amiodarone was associated with a 2% rate of hyperthyroidism. In contrast, in Pisa, Italy, an area of borderline iodine intake and a high prevalence of nodular goiter, amiodarone was associated with 9.6% rate of hyperthyroidism [67].

The clinical effects of amiodarone on thyroid function in any individual are dependent upon the underlying status of that individual's thyroid gland. In euthyroid individuals receiving amiodarone, acute changes in thyroid function tests include [68, 69]:

- Serum total T4 and free T4 concentrations rise by 20–40% during the first month of therapy.

- Serum T3 concentrations decrease by up to 30% within the first few weeks of therapy.

- Serum rT3 concentrations increase by 20% soon after the initiation of therapy.

- Serum TSH concentration usually rises slightly after the initiation of treatment and may exceed the upper limit of normal.

After 3–6 months of therapy, a steady state is reached in most patients who were euthyroid at baseline:

- Serum TSH concentration normalizes.

- Serum total T4, free T4, and rT3 concentrations remain slightly elevated or in the upper normal range.

- Serum T3 concentrations remain in the low normal range.

Amiodarone may also cause destructive thyroiditis with transient thyrotoxicosis followed by hypothyroidism in patients without underlying thyroid disease [60].

Abnormal thyroid process: in patients with underlying multinodular goiter or latent Graves' disease, hyperthyroidism (increased synthesis of T4 and T3) may occur. The excess iodine from the amiodarone provides increased substrate, resulting in enhanced thyroid hormone production.

3.4.4 Clinical forms of amiodarone-induced hyperthyroidism

Three types of AIT can be distinguished. In type 1 AIT, thyroid hormone synthesis is increased, whereas in type 2 there is an excess release of T4 and T3 from the preformed thyroid hormones, due to destructive thyroiditis. Type 3 AIT is a mixed form, existing an overlapping condition between type 1 and type 2 AIT. These types differ in their pathogenesis, clinical or paraclinical signs, and management [63].

The risk of either type increases with higher cumulative doses or reintroduction of amiodarone [53, 70].

The distribution of AIT by type (1 or 2) varies by geographical region. This is thought to be primarily due to differences in dietary iodine intake. In iodine-deficient regions, as some geographical zones were in Romania before universal salt iodization [3], AIT occurs in approximately 10–12% of patients with type 1 AIT usually predominating [64, 67]. However, the distribution of cases by type may be changing, as illustrated in a report of 215 consecutive patients with AIT seen at a single institution in Italy over 26 years [71]. In 1980 compared with 2006, 2 of 6 (40%) versus 12 of 14 (86%) of new AIT cases were type 2. Possible explanations for this observation include improved dietary iodine intake in the region and the avoidance of amiodarone use in case of previously diagnosed thyroid disease. Our unpublished data from a study conducted in a single institute (Endocrinology Clinic, Târgu Mureş, Romania) in two different periods, which included 5 years, similarly show a moderate increase of type 2 AIT after the introduction of universal salt iodization (governmental decision no. 586/5 June 2002; see **Table 4**).

Clinical signs of AIT are classical thyrotoxicosis symptoms such as unexplained weight loss, proximal myopathy, restlessness, heat intolerance, low-grade fever, or exacerbation of tachyarrhythmia, heart failure, or angina pectoris; however, the adrenergic manifestations of amiodarone-induced hyperthyroidism are often masked because its distinct antiadrenergic properties and impairment of conversion of T4 to T3 [68, 72]. Patients with amiodarone-induced hyperthyroidism have a threefold higher rate of major adverse cardiovascular events (mostly ventricular arrhythmias) compared with euthyroid controls [73]. The presence of severe left ventricular dysfunction, especially in older patients with AIT, may be associated with increased mortality [74].

Differentiating the two types of AIT is critical since therapy differs. However, the distinction may be difficult using clinical criteria, partly because some patients may have a mixture of both mechanisms, presenting the type 3 (type 1 + type 2) AIT. Thyroid function tests (TSH, T4 and T3 plasma levels) do not help to distinguish type 1 AIT (hyperthyroidism) from type 2 AIT (transient thyrotoxicosis).

Type 1 AIT appears usually early after amiodarone introduction (3–20 months after exposure) [19, 66, 71]. It is characterized by hyperfunctional thyroid tissue with elevated blood flow on color Doppler [75, 76]. Furthermore, the enlarged or nodular thyroid tissue fixes either on 24-hour 123I-scan or on 99 mTc-SestaMIBI radio isotope scan despite the daily ingestion of 6 mg or more bioavailable iodine [77, 78].

Study period	Type 1 AIT/total patients	Type 2 AIT/total patients	Type 3 AIT/total patients
1994–1998	4/7 (57%)	1/7 (14%)	2/7 (29%)
2001–2005	17/38 (45%)	9/38(24%)	12/38 (31%)

Table 4.
Distribution of AIT types in patients of the Endocrinology Clinic, Târgu Mureş, Romania, in two study periods (1994–1998 and 2001–2005).

	Type 1 AIT	Type 2 AIT
Pre-existing thyroid disease	Yes	No
Pathophysiology	Iodine overload	Destruction/inflammation
Ultrasound findings	Goiter/nodule(s)	Normal
Color flow Doppler	Increased or vascularity	Reduced or absent vascularity
Radio iodine uptake (I123-Scan)/ SestaMIBI-Scan	Normal or increased	Absent

Table 5.
Characteristics of type 1 and type 2 amiodarone-induced thyrotoxicosis (AIT—amiodarone-induced thyrotoxicosis).

Type 2 AIT is a destructive thyroiditis which onset time is after 20–30 months of amiodarone introduction. It appears in patients with apparently normal thyroid morphology and is due to the massive release of thyroid hormones. The mechanism is similar to that of subacute thyroiditis, but the thyrotoxicosis is usually less severe and could spontaneously resolve in some cases [79]. The features of the two types of AIT are presented in **Table 5**.

However, interpretations of color flow Doppler sonogram in amiodarone-associated hyperthyroidism require an experienced sonographer, and other markers for differential diagnosis were also sought. In two studies, serum interleukin-6 concentrations were higher in patients with type 2 AIT [80, 81]. In a third study, interleukin-6 concentrations were not useful for distinguishing type 1 from type 2 AIT [76].

4. Prevention and treatment of iodine-induced thyrotoxicosis

Preventing therapy for iodine-induced hyperthyroidism is not generally recommended. However, older patients with known multinodular goiter and/or subclinical hyperthyroidism should be told of the risk for iodine-induced hyperthyroidism, and alternatives to contrast-enhanced CT scanning should be considered when appropriate (e.g., noncontrast CT, magnetic resonance imaging). Iodine-induced hyperthyroidism is particularly important in geriatric patients for several reasons: (1) the prevalence of thyroid nodular disease is higher in older patients than in younger patients, (2) the hyperthyroidism may be more difficult to detect clinically, (3) apathetic hyperthyroidism often being present, and (4) older adults more often have underlying heart disease [21]. In high-risk patients (older, history of multinodular goiter with autonomy), treatment with a thioamide or perchlorate prior to the administration of an iodine load may blunt or prevent the induction of hyperthyroidism [82, 83]. However, there are insufficient randomized trial data to support the use of thioamides or perchlorate. Routine measurement of thyroid function tests (TSH, and if low, free T4 and T3) in older patients after exposure to iodinated radiographic contrast agents is favored by some experts, particularly since the symptoms of hyperthyroidism in older adults may be atypical [84–86].

Iodine-induced hyperthyroidism (iodine content supplements and dietary nutrients, ICM, type 1 AIT) is usually self-limited (lasting 1–18 months) if the source of iodine is discontinued. The American Thyroid Association (ATA) [87] and European Thyroid Association (ETA) recommendations [40] as initial therapy for patients with iodine-induced hyperthyroidism are discontinuation of iodine (except for amiodarone, which could be continued in type 2 AIT), avoidance of further exposure, and administration of a beta-adrenergic antagonist drug (assuming there are no contraindications to its use) to minimize the manifestations of the overactive thyroid. Thyroid tests (TSH, free T4, total T3) should be measured initially at 4- to 6-week interval and then less frequently (TSH and free T4 every 3 months) depending upon the results of prior testing. Beta blockers can be tapered and discontinued after thyroid tests return to normal.

Due to the lack of sufficient evidence, there is no consensus regarding the decision to continue or stop amiodarone in patients with type 1 AIT. The decision should be individualized taking into account the risks of patients and taken jointly by cardiologists and endocrinologist [40]. Amiodarone should be continued in critically ill patients with life-threatening cardiac disorders [88]. When deciding whether to discontinue amiodarone, the following should be considered: amiodarone may be necessary to control a life-threatening arrhythmia; since the half-life of elimination from the body is prolonged, there is no immediate benefit to stopping amiodarone; amiodarone appears to ameliorate hyperthyroidism by blocking T4 to T3 conversion, beta-adrenergic receptors, and possibly T3 receptors. Stopping amiodarone might actually exacerbate hyperthyroid symptoms and signs.

In case of amiodarone withdrawal, after the restoration of euthyroidism and normalization of urinary iodine excretion (generally 6–12 months), radioactive iodine (RAI) therapy can be performed. Recombinant human TSH (rhTSH) administration increases the sensibility of the thyroid gland to RAI therapy. If RAI administration is contraindicated, total thyroidectomy should be considered for definitive treatment of the underlying thyroid disease [40]. In the absence of the thyroid gland, amiodarone reintroduction, when necessary, could be safe. In the case of the thyroid gland is conserved, the recurrence rate of type 1 AIT after amiodarone reintroduction is 9% [89]. As ETA suggested, emergency thyroidectomy in severe cardiac patients may be required not only in type 1 but also in all types of AIT. Prior to thyroid surgery, plasmapheresis is able to remove the excess of thyroid hormones [40]. It was reported in a study, including seven patients with AIT, that iopanoic acid short-course administration prior surgery permitted a safe and uneventful thyroidectomy [90].

Thioamides (thiamazole, carbimazole, propylthiouracil) are effective in older patients with underlying heart disease having severe and prolonged (>1 month) hyperthyroid symptoms, except the emergency situations. All thioamides are blocking thyroid hormones synthesis, propylthiouracil having an additional inhibiting effect on T4–T3 transformation. ATA recommended, the starting dose of thiamazole, to be 10–20 mg once daily because of its long duration of action, allowing for once-daily dosing, more rapid efficacy, and lower incidence of side effects [87]. ETA recommended very high daily doses of the drug (40–60 mg/day of thiamazole) for a more extended time, considering that in type 1 AIT the iodine-enriched thyroid gland of patients is less responsive to thioamides [40]. Carbimazole, the prodrug of thiamazole, is an alternative choice of treatment, available in some European countries, but not in Romania. Due to the teratogenicity of thiamazole, propylthiouracil (not currently available in Romania) can be used in the first trimester of pregnancy [68]. To increase the sensitivity and response of the thyroid gland to thioamides, potassium or sodium perchlorate (not available in Romania) has been used. Perchlorate reduces thyroid iodine uptake by sodium/iodide symporter inhibiting action and discharge iodine from the thyroid, but toxic effects are limiting its use. To minimize the nephro- and medullotoxicity of the drug, doses not exceeding 4×250 mg/day and a shorter period than 4–6 weeks were used [40, 87, 91]. Thyroid function should be assessed after 4 weeks by measurement of serum TSH, free T4, and T3. The dose of thiamazole is then tapered with the goal of maintaining a euthyroid state. Thereafter, thyroid function tests (TSH, free T4) should be measured every 3 months. Many patients with underlying autonomous nodular thyroid disease are able to taper and discontinue thiamazole within 6–12 months. In case of thioamide allergy, lithium is used to control the hyperthyroidism temporarily [91, 92], but it has a narrow therapeutic range, produces nephrotoxicity, and its efficacy is not well documented. Therefore, it is not recommended by ETA for the type 1 AIT treatment [40]. However, it was reported that lithium-associated rhTSH administration increases RAI sensibility of the thyroid follicles in AIT [93].

After resolution of the acute episode of iodine-induced hyperthyroidism, treatment of the underlying thyroid disease should be addressed. For patients with underlying Graves' disease, treatment options include continuing thiamazole, radioiodine ablation, or surgery. Patients with underlying autonomous adenoma or multinodular goiter who return to euthyroidism after discontinuation of iodine do not necessarily require definitive treatment. However, these patients are at risk for recurrent hyperthyroidism if given iodine again.

Type 2 AIT generally is self-limited and amiodarone is not necessary to discontinue. When the efficacy of non-thioamide type antithyroid drugs to restore euthyroid state was compared, the best results were obtained with 30 mg oral prednisone therapy. The rate of achievement of euthyroid state was 100% when glucocorticoids were used versus 71% obtained after perchlorate administration [94]. ETA recommendation, for this reason, is oral glucocorticoids as the first-line treatment for type 2 AIT. In patients in whom a mixed form of AIT is suspected, thioamides together with glucocorticoids should be given initially, or glucocorticoids should be added after a period of 4–6 weeks of inadequate response [40]. In addition, it must be noted that i.v. administration of glucocorticoids (hydrocortisone, dexamethasone) has crucial benefits (inhibiting T4 transformation to T3) in thyroid storm and preoperative management of any type of thyrotoxicosis [91]. It was reported that glucocorticoid therapy (oral prednisone) restored the normal thyroid function and shrink goiter, preventing surgery, in a patient diagnosed with iodine containing supplement-induced hyperthyroidism [95].

5. Conclusions

Iodine, as an essential microelement of the human body, plays a very important role in thyroid physiology. Adequate intake is necessary to keep thyroid hormone synthesis at normal rate. Dietary intake and urinary excretion should be equivalent, but a remarkable adaptive capacity of the thyroid gland can compensate for excess intake on short term. However, existing thyroid disease (subclinical or overt) or specific risk factors may impair the patient's response to high iodine exposure, which can result in hypothyroidism or hyperthyroidism. On the other hand, iodine excess may also be hardly recognizable because various sources (e.g. seafood, kelp, dairy products, iodized salt, iodized water, nutritional supplements, iodine containing contrast media, and drugs) can all contribute to iodine intake. Of these, iodine containing contrast media and drugs are administered only under controlled conditions but represent the most frequent cause of iodine-induced thyrotoxicosis. In general, preventive actions are not recommended, but screening for risk factors, such as elderly patients, persons with multinodular goiter, subclinical hyperthyroidism, or manifest hyperthyroidism should take place prior to iodine administration. Consequently, high-risk patients should benefit preventive treatment with thioamide or perchlorate. Amiodarone-induced thyrotoxicosis has remained a difficult task requiring a close collaboration between cardiology and endocrinology to overcome complications, but individualization of the therapy should be undertaken. Based on the specific features of thyrotoxicosis, thioamides, perchlorate, or high-dose glucocorticoids may be considered for an optimal therapeutic intervention. If contraindicated, radioiodine therapy may also be useful to treat amiodarone-induced thyrotoxicosis.

Conflict of interest

The authors declare no conflict of interest.

Abbreviations

AIT	amiodarone-induced thyrotoxicosis
ATA	American Thyroid Association
CT	computed tomography
DEA	N-desethylamiodarone
ETA	European Thyroid Association
ICM	iodinated contrast media
MUIC	median urinary iodine content
RAI	radioactive iodine
RDA	recommended daily allowances
rhTSH	recombinant human thyroid stimulating hormone
rT3	reverse 3,3′,5′-triiodothyronine
T3	3,5,3′-triiodothyronine
T4	thyroxine
TSH	thyroid stimulating hormone
WHO	World Health Organization

Author details

Melinda Kolcsár and Zsolt Gáll*
University of Medicine, Pharmacy, Sciences and Technology of Târgu Mureș, Romania

*Address all correspondence to: zsolt.gall@umfst.ro

References

[1] Andersson M, de Benoist B, Delange F, Zupan J, Zupan J. Prevention and control of iodine deficiency in pregnant and lactating women and in children less than 2-years-old: Conclusions and recommendations of the technical consultation. Public Health Nutrition. 2007;**10**:1606-1611

[2] Iodine Global Network (IGN)—Romania [Internet]. 2019. Available from: http://www.ign.org/p142001976.html [Accessed: 18 July 2019]

[3] Kun IZ, Szántó Z, Balázs J, Năsălean A, Gliga C. Detection of iodine deficiency disorders (goiter and hypothyroidism) in school-children living in endemic mountainous regions, after the implementation of universal salt iodization. In: Hot Top. Endocr. Endocrine-Related Dis. Rijeka, Croatia: IntechOpen; 2013. DOI: 10.5772/54188

[4] Roti E, Uberti ED. Iodine excess and hyperthyroidism. Thyroid. 2001;**11**:493-500. DOI: 10.1089/105072501300176453

[5] Abel MH, Korevaar TIM, Erlund I, Villanger GD, Caspersen IH, Arohonka P, et al. Iodine intake is associated with thyroid function in mild to moderately iodine deficient pregnant women. Thyroid. 2018;**28**:1359-1371. DOI: 10.1089/thy.2018.0305

[6] Wolff J, Chaikoff IL. Plasma inorganic iodide as a homeostatic regulator of thyroid function. The Journal of Biological Chemistry. 1948;**174**:555-564

[7] Scientific Opinion on Dietary Reference Values for Iodine. EFSA J [Internet]. 2014. p. 12. Available from: https://efsa.onlinelibrary.wiley.com/doi/pdf/10.2903/j.efsa.2014.3660 [Accessed: 18 July 2019]

[8] Allain P, Berre S, Krari N, Lainé-Cessac P, Le Bouil A, Barbot N, et al. Use of plasma iodine assay for diagnosing thyroid disorders. Journal of Clinical Pathology. 1993;**46**:453-455. DOI: 10.1136/jcp.46.5.453

[9] Michalke B, Schramel P, Witte H. Iodine speciation in human serum by reversed-phase liquid chromatography-ICP-mass spectrometry. Biological Trace Element Research. 2000;**78**:81-92. DOI: 10.1385/BTER:78:1-3:81

[10] Farebrother J, Zimmermann MB, Andersson M. Excess iodine intake: Sources, assessment, and effects on thyroid function. Annals of the New York Academy of Sciences. 2019;**1446**(1):44-65. DOI: 10.1111/nyas.14041

[11] Zhao J, Wang P, Shang L, Sullivan KM, van der Haar F, Maberly G. Endemic goiter associated with high iodine intake. American Journal of Public Health. 2000;**90**:1633-1635. DOI: 10.2105/ajph.90.10.1633

[12] Teng W, Shan Z, Teng X, Guan H, Li Y, Teng D, et al. Effect of iodine intake on thyroid diseases in China. The New England Journal of Medicine. 2006;**354**:2783-2793. DOI: 10.1056/NEJMoa054022

[13] Katagiri R, Yuan X, Kobayashi S, Sasaki S. Effect of excess iodine intake on thyroid diseases in different populations: A systematic review and meta-analyses including observational studies. PLoS One. 2017;**12**:e0173722. DOI: 10.1371/journal.pone.0173722

[14] Mancini FR, Rajaobelina K, Dow C, Habbal T, Affret A, Balkau B, et al. High iodine dietary intake is associated with type 2 diabetes among women of the E3N-EPIC cohort study. Clinical Nutrition. 2019;**38**:1651-1656. DOI: 10.1016/j.clnu.2018.08.015

[15] Delange F, de Benoist B, Alnwick D. Risks of iodine-induced hyperthyroidism after correction of iodine deficiency by iodized salt. Thyroid. 1999;**9**:545-556. DOI: 10.1089/thy.1999.9.545

[16] Laurberg P, Cerqueira C, Ovesen L, Rasmussen LB, Perrild H, Andersen S, et al. Iodine intake as a determinant of thyroid disorders in populations. Best Practice & Research Clinical Endocrinology & Metabolism. 2010;**24**:13-27. DOI: 10.1016/j.beem.2009.08.013

[17] Kahaly GJ, Dienes HP, Beyer J, Hommel G. Iodide induces thyroid autoimmunity in patients with endemic goitre: A randomised, double-blind, placebo-controlled trial. European Journal of Endocrinology. 1998;**139**:290-297

[18] Rabinowe SL, Larsen PR, Antman EM, George KL, Friedman PL, Jackson RA, et al. Amiodarone therapy and autoimmune thyroid disease: Increase in a new monoclonal antibody-defined T cell subset. The American Journal of Medicine. 1986;**81**:53-57. DOI: 10.1016/0002-9343(86)90181-6

[19] Martino E, Bartalena L, Bogazzi F, Braverman LE. The effects of amiodarone on the thyroid. Endocrine Reviews. 2001;**22**(2): 240-254. DOI: 10.1210/edrv.22.2.0427

[20] World Health Organization. Salt as a Vehicle for Fortification. Report of a WHO Expert Consultation [Internet]. Luxembourg: World Health Organization; 2008. Available from: https://apps.who.int/iris/handle/10665/43908 [Accessed: 18 July 2019]

[21] Stanbury JB, Ermans AE, Bourdoux P, Todd C, Oken E, Tonglet R, et al. Iodine-induced hyperthyroidism: Occurrence and epidemiology. Thyroid. 1998;**8**:83-100. DOI: 10.1089/thy.1998.8.83

[22] Parveen S, Latif SA, Kamal MM, Asaduzzaman M, Akther A, Laila ZH. Iodized salt induced thyrotoxicosis: Bangladesh perspective. Mymensingh Medical Journal. 2009;**18**:165-168

[23] Leung AM. The effects of iodine excess. In: Pearce EN, editor. Iodine Deficiency Disorders and Their Elimination. Cham: Springer International Publishing; 2017. pp. 75-89. DOI: 10.1007/978-3-319-49505-7_6

[24] Leung AM, Braverman LE. Consequences of excess iodine. Nature Reviews Endocrinology. 2014;**10**: 136-142. DOI: 10.1038/nrendo.2013.251

[25] Choudhry H, Nasrullah M. Iodine consumption and cognitive performance: Confirmation of adequate consumption. Food Science. 2018;**6**:1341-1351. DOI: 10.1002/fsn3.694

[26] Taylor T, Czarnowski C. What caused this case of asymptomatic hyperthyroidism? Everything pointed to an exogenous cause, but our patient denied taking anything. Only later did she mention a diet aid. The Journal of Family Practice. 2009;**58**:203-207

[27] Taylor JE, Fishman SL, Morris M, Krymskaya M, Goldman R, Poretsky L. A case of hyperthyroidism in a patient using the nutritional supplement "survival shield". AACE Clinical Case Reports. 2018;**4**:e398-e401. DOI: 10.4158/ACCR-2018-0086

[28] Shilo S, Hirsch HJ. Iodine-induced hyperthyroidism in a patient with a normal thyroid gland. Postgraduate Medical Journal. 1986;**62**:661-662. DOI: 10.1136/pgmj.62.729.661

[29] Clark CD, Bassett B, Burge MR. Effects of kelp supplementation on

thyroid function in euthyroid subjects. Endocrine Practice. 2003;**9**:363-369. DOI: 10.4158/EP.9.5.363

[30] Di Matola T, Zeppa P, Gasperi M, Vitale M. Thyroid dysfunction following a kelp-containing marketed diet. BML Case Reports. 2014;**pii**:bcr2014206330. DOI: 10.1136/bcr-2014-206330

[31] ACR Manual On Contrast Media [Internet]. 2018. Available from: https://www.acr.org/-/media/ACR/Files/Clinical-Resources/Contrast_Media.pdf [Accessed: 01 August 2019]

[32] Solomon R, Biguori C, Bettmann M. Selection of contrast media. Kidney International. 2006;**69**:S39-S45. DOI: 10.1038/sj.ki.5000373

[33] The Royal Australian and New Zealand College of Radiologists. Iodinated Contrast Media Guideline V2.3 [Internet]. 2018. Available from: https://www.ranzcr.com/college/document-library/ranzcr-iodinated-contrast-guidelines [Accessed: 01 August 2019]

[34] Nouh MR, El-Shazly MA. Radiographic and magnetic resonances contrast agents: Essentials and tips for safe practices. World Journal of Radiology. 2017;**9**:339-349. DOI: 10.4329/wjr.v9.i9.339

[35] Thomsen HS, European Society of Urogenital Radiology. European Society of Urogenital Radiology guidelines on contrast media application. Current Opinion in Urology. 2007;**17**:70-76. DOI: 10.1097/MOU.0b013e328011c96f

[36] van der Molen AJ, Thomsen HS, Morcos SK, Almén T, Aspelin P, Bellin MF, et al. Effect of iodinated contrast media on thyroid function in adults. European Radiology. 2004;**14**:902-907. DOI: 10.1007/s00330-004-2238-z

[37] Lee SY, Rhee CM, Leung AM, Braverman LE, Brent GA, Pearce EN. A review: Radiographic iodinated contrast media-induced thyroid dysfunction. The Journal of Clinical Endocrinology and Metabolism. 2015;**100**:376-383. DOI: 10.1210/jc.2014-3292

[38] Gartner W, Weissel M. Do iodine-containing contrast media induce clinically relevant changes in thyroid function parameters of euthyroid patients within the first week? Thyroid. 2004;**14**:521-524. DOI: 10.1089/1050725041517075

[39] Kornelius E, Chiou J-Y, Yang Y-S, Lo S-C, Peng C-H, Lai Y-R, et al. Iodinated contrast media–induced thyroid dysfunction in euthyroid nodular goiter patients. Thyroid. 2016;**26**:1030-1038. DOI: 10.1089/thy.2016.0051

[40] Bartalena L, Bogazzi F, Chiovato L, Hubalewska-Dydejczyk A, Links TP, Vanderpump M. 2018 European thyroid association (ETA) guidelines for the management of amiodarone-associated thyroid dysfunction. European Thyroid Journal. 2018;**7**:55-66. DOI: 10.1159/000486957

[41] Ahmet A, Lawson ML, Babyn P, Tricco AC. Hypothyroidism in neonates post-iodinated contrast media: A systematic review. Acta Paediatrica. 2009;**98**:1568-1574. DOI: 10.1111/j.1651-2227.2009.01412.x

[42] Kornelius E, Chiou J-Y, Yang Y-S, Peng C-H, Lai Y-R, Huang C-N. Iodinated contrast media increased the risk of thyroid dysfunction: A 6-year retrospective cohort study. The Journal of Clinical Endocrinology and Metabolism. 2015;**100**:3372-3379. DOI: 10.1210/JC.2015-2329

[43] Rhee CM, Bhan I, Alexander EK, Brunelli SM. Association between iodinated contrast media exposure and incident hyperthyroidism and

hypothyroidism. Archives of Internal Medicine. 2012;**172**:153. DOI: 10.1001/archinternmed.2011.677

[44] Kodama I, Kamiya K, Toyama J. Amiodarone: Ionic and cellular mechanisms of action of the most promising class III agent. The American Journal of Cardiology. 1999;**84**:20R-28R. DOI: 10.1016/s0002-9149(99)00698-0

[45] Latini R, Tognoni G, Kates RE. Clinical pharmacokinetics of amiodarone. Clinical Pharmacokinetics. 1984;**9**:136-156. DOI: 10.2165/00003088-198409020-00002

[46] van der Haar F, Gerasimov G, Tyler VQ, Timmer A. Universal salt iodization in the central and Eastern Europe, commonwealth of independent states (CEE/CIS) region during the decade 2000-09: Experiences, achievements, and lessons learned. Food and Nutrition Bulletin. 2011;**32**(4 Suppl):S175-S294. DOI: 10.1177/15648265110324S401

[47] Lazarus JH. Iodine Status in Europe in 2014. European Thyroid Journal. 2014;**3**:3-6. DOI: 10.1159/000358873

[48] Zhou L, Chen BP, Kluger J, Fan C, Chow MS. Effects of amiodarone and its active metabolite desethylamiodarone on the ventricular defibrillation threshold. Journal of the American College of Cardiology. 1998;**31**:1672-1678. DOI: 10.1016/s0735-1097(98)00160-0

[49] Rotmensch HH, Belhassen B, Swanson BN, Shoshani D, Spielman SR, Greenspon AJ, et al. Steady-state serum amiodarone concentrations: Relationships with antiarrhythmic efficacy and toxicity. Annals of Internal Medicine. 1984;**101**:462. DOI: 10.7326/0003-4819-101-4-462

[50] Campbell TJ, Williams KM. Therapeutic drug monitoring: Antiarrhythmic drugs. British Journal of Clinical Pharmacology. 2001;**52**(Suppl 1):21S-34S. DOI: 10.1046/j.1365-2125.2001.0520s1021.x

[51] Hofmann A, Nawara C, Ofluoglu S, Holzmannhofer J, Strohmer B, Pirich C. Incidence and predictability of amiodarone-induced thyrotoxicosis and hypothyroidism. Wiener klinische Wochenschrift. 2008;**120**:493-498. DOI: 10.1007/s00508-008-1017-2

[52] Ahmed S, Van Gelder IC, Wiesfeld ACP, Van Veldhuisen DJ, Links TP. Determinants and outcome of amiodarone-associated thyroid dysfunction. Clinical Endocrinology. 2011;**75**:388-394. DOI: 10.1111/j.1365-2265.2011.04087.x

[53] Bouvy ML, Heerdink ER, Hoes AW, Leufkens HGM. Amiodarone-induced thyroid dysfunction associated with cumulative dose. Pharmacoepidemiology and Drug Safety. 2002;**11**:601-606. DOI: 10.1002/pds.735

[54] Ross ADS. Amiodarone and Thyroid Dysfunction [Internet]. 2019. Available from: https://www.uptodate.com/contents/amiodarone-and-thyroid-dysfunction [Accessed: 18 July 2018]

[55] Mosher MC. Amiodarone-induced hypothyroidism and other adverse effects. Dimensions of Critical Care Nursing. 2011;**30**:87-93. DOI: 10.1097/DCC.0b013e3182052130

[56] Eng PH, Cardona GR, Fang SL, Previti M, Alex S, Carrasco N, et al. Escape from the acute Wolff-Chaikoff effect is associated with a decrease in thyroid sodium/iodide symporter messenger ribonucleic acid and protein. Endocrinology. 1999;**140**:3404-3410. DOI: 10.1210/endo.140.8.6893

[57] Vagenakis AG, Braverman LE. Drug induced hypothyroidism. Pharmacology

& Therapeutics. Part C: Clinical Pharmacology and Therapeutics. 1976;**1**:149-159. DOI: 10.1016/S0362-5486(76)80011-8

[58] van Beeren HC, Bakker O, Wiersinga WM. Desethylamiodarone is a competitive inhibitor of the binding of thyroid hormone to the thyroid hormone α1-receptor protein. Molecular and Cellular Endocrinology. 1995;**112**:15-19

[59] Bogazzi F, Bartalena L, Brogioni S, Burelli A, Raggi F, Ultimieri F, et al. Desethylamiodarone antagonizes the effect of thyroid hormone at the molecular level. European Journal of Endocrinology. 2001;**145**:59-64

[60] Roti E, Minelli R, Gardini E, Bianconi L, Braverman LE. Thyrotoxicosis followed by hypothyroidism in patients treated with amiodarone. Archives of Internal Medicine. 1993;**153**:886

[61] Aleksić Ž, Aleksić A, Mitov V, Jović M, Zdravković D. Amiodarone treatment and thyroid autoimmunity markers. Hellenic Journal of Nuclear Medicine. 2008;**11**:105-109

[62] Danzi S, Klein I. Amiodarone-induced thyroid dysfunction. Journal of Intensive Care Medicine. 2015;**30**:179-185. DOI: 10.1177/0885066613503278

[63] Maqdasy S, Benichou T, Dallel S, Roche B, Desbiez F, Montanier N, et al. Issues in amiodarone-induced thyrotoxicosis: Update and review of the literature. Annales d'Endocrinologie. 2019;**80**:54-60. DOI: 10.1016/j.ando.2018.05.001

[64] Trip MD, Wiersinga W, Plomp TA. Incidence, predictability, and pathogenesis of amiodarone-induced thyrotoxicosis and hypothyroidism. The American Journal of Medicine. 1991;**91**:507-511. DOI: 10.1016/0002-9343(91)90187-3

[65] Sidhu J, Jenkins D. Men are at increased risk of amiodarone-associated thyrotoxicosis in the UK. QJM: An International Journal of Medicine. 2003;**96**:949-950. DOI: 10.1093/qjmed/hcg158

[66] Tomisti L, Rossi G, Bartalena L, Martino E, Bogazzi F. The onset time of amiodarone-induced thyrotoxicosis (AIT) depends on AIT type. European Journal of Endocrinology. 2014;**171**: 363-368. DOI: 10.1530/EJE-14-0267

[67] Martino E. Environmental iodine intake and thyroid dysfunction during chronic amiodarone therapy. Annals of Internal Medicine. 1984;**101**:28-34. DOI: 10.7326/0003-4819-101-1-28

[68] Basaria S, Cooper DS. Amiodarone and the thyroid. The American Journal of Medicine. 2005;**118**:706-714. DOI: 10.1016/j.amjmed.2004.11.028

[69] Diederichsen SZ, Darkner S, Chen X, Johannesen A, Pehrson S, Hansen J, et al. Short-term amiodarone treatment for atrial fibrillation after catheter ablation induces a transient thyroid dysfunction: Results from the placebo-controlled, randomized AMIO-CAT trial. European Journal of Internal Medicine. 2016;**33**:36-41. DOI: 10.1016/j.ejim.2016.04.012

[70] Maqdasy S, Batisse-Lignier M, Auclair C, Desbiez F, Citron B, Thieblot P, et al. Amiodarone-induced thyrotoxicosis recurrence after amiodarone reintroduction. The American Journal of Cardiology. 2016;**117**:1112-1116. DOI: 10.1016/j.amjcard.2016.01.003

[71] Bogazzi F, Bartalena L, Dell'Unto E, Tomisti L, Rossi G, Pepe P, et al. Proportion of type 1 and type 2 amiodarone-induced thyrotoxicosis has changed over a 27-year period in Italy. Clinical Endocrinology. 2007;**67**(4):533-537. DOI: 10.1111/j.1365-2265.2007.02920.x

[72] Ghuran AV, Camm AJ. Amiodarone and beta blockade amiodarone and beta blockade-is the whole better than parts? Journal of Clinical and Basic Cardiology. 2000;**3**(3):205-207

[73] Yiu K-H, Jim M-H, Siu C-W, Lee C-H, Yuen M, Mok M, et al. Amiodarone-induced thyrotoxicosis is a predictor of adverse cardiovascular outcome. The Journal of Clinical Endocrinology and Metabolism. 2009;**94**:109-114. DOI: 10.1210/jc.2008-1907

[74] O'Sullivan AJ, Lewis M, Diamond T. Amiodarone-induced thyrotoxicosis: Left ventricular dysfunction is associated with increased mortality. European Journal of Endocrinology. 2006;**154**:533-536. DOI: 10.1530/eje.1.02122

[75] Bogazzi F, Bartalena L, Brogioni S, Mazzeo S, Vitti P, Burelli A, et al. Color flow Doppler sonography rapidly differentiates type I and type II amiodarone-induced thyrotoxicosis. Thyroid. 1997;7:541-545. DOI: 10.1089/thy.1997.7.541

[76] Eaton SEM, Euinton HA, Newman CM, Weetman AP, Bennet WM. Clinical experience of amiodarone-induced thyrotoxicosis over a 3-year period: Role of colour-flow Doppler sonography. Clinical Endocrinology. 2002;**56**:33-38

[77] Patel NR, Tamara LA, Lee H. 99mTc sestamibi thyroid scan in amiodarone-induced thyrotoxicosis type I. Clinical Nuclear Medicine. 2016;**41**:566-567. DOI: 10.1097/RLU.0000000000001243

[78] Bogazzi F, Martino E, Dell'Unto E, Brogioni S, Cosci C, Aghini-Lombardi F, et al. Thyroid color flow Doppler sonography and radioiodine uptake in 55 consecutive patients with amiodarone-induced thyrotoxicosis. Journal of Endocrinological Investigation. 2003;**26**:635-640. DOI: 10.1007/BF03347021

[79] Osman F, Franklyn JA, Sheppard MC, Gammage MD. Successful treatment of amiodarone-induced thyrotoxicosis. Circulation. 2002;**105**:1275-1277. DOI: 10.1161/circ.105.11.1275

[80] Bartalena L, Brogioni S, Grasso L, Bogazzi F, Burelli A, Martino E. Treatment of amiodarone-induced thyrotoxicosis, a difficult challenge: Results of a prospective study. The Journal of Clinical Endocrinology and Metabolism. 1996;**81**(8):2930-2933. DOI: 10.1210/jcem.81.8.8768854

[81] Bartalena L, Grasso L, Brogioni S, Aghini-Lombardi F, Braverman LE, Martino E. Serum interleukin-6 in amiodarone-induced thyrotoxicosis. The Journal of Clinical Endocrinology and Metabolism. 1994;**78**:423-427. DOI: 10.1210/jcem.78.2.8106631

[82] Nolte, Muller R, Siggelkow H, Emrich D, Hufner M. Prophylactic application of thyrostatic drugs during excessive iodine exposure in euthyroid patients with thyroid autonomy: A randomized study. European Journal of Endocrinology. 1996;**134**:337-341

[83] Lawrence JE, Lamm SH, Braverman LE. The use of perchlorate for the prevention of thyrotoxicosis in patients given iodine rich contrast agents. Journal of Endocrinological Investigation. 1999;**22**:405-407. DOI: 10.1007/BF03343581

[84] Torre R, Del Monte P, Bernasconi D, Marugo A, Poggi P, Leoncini R, et al. Screening for thyroid disorders in elderly patients. Recenti Progressi in Medicina. 2004;**95**:308-311

[85] Rozendaal FP. Hyperthyroidism in the elderly: A specific signs may cause a delay in diagnosis. Tijdschrift voor Gerontologie en Geriatrie. 2005;**36**:77-80

[86] Martin FI, Deam DR. Hyperthyroidism in elderly hospitalised patients. Clinical features and treatment outcomes. The Medical Journal of Australia. 1996;**164**:200-203

[87] Bahn RS, Burch HB, Cooper DS, Garber JR, Greenlee MC, Klein I, et al. Hyperthyroidism and other causes of thyrotoxicosis: Management guidelines of the American Thyroid Association and American Association of Clinical Endocrinologists. Thyroid. 2011;**21**:593-646. DOI: 10.1089/thy.2010.0417

[88] Tauveron I, Batisse-Lignier M, Maqdasy S. Challenges in the management of amiodarone-induced thyrotoxicosis. Presse Médicale. 2018;**47**:746-756. DOI: 10.1016/j.lpm.2018.09.001

[89] Ryan LE, Braverman LE, Cooper DS, Ladenson PW, Kloos RT. Can amiodarone be restarted after amiodarone-induced thyrotoxicosis? Thyroid. 2004;**14**:149-153. DOI: 10.1089/105072504322880391

[90] Bogazzi F, Miccoli P, Berti P, Cosci C, Brogioni S, Aghini-Lombardi F, et al. Preparation with iopanoic acid rapidly controls thyrotoxicosis in patients with amiodarone-induced thyrotoxicosis before thyroidectomy. Surgery. 2002;**132**:1114-1118. DOI: 10.1067/msy.2002.128561

[91] Suwansaksri N, Preechasuk L, Kunavisarut T. Nonthionamide drugs for the treatment of hyperthyroidism: From present to future. International Journal of Endocrinology. 2018;**2018**:1-10. DOI: 10.1155/2018/5794054

[92] Dickstein G, Shechner C, Adawi F, Kaplan J, Baron E, Ish-Shalom S. Lithium treatment in amiodarone-induced thyrotoxicosis. The American Journal of Medicine. 1997;**102**:454-458. DOI: 10.1016/S0002-9343(97)00047-8

[93] Laplano NER, Mercado-Asis LB. Recombinant TSH and lithium overcomes amiodarone-induced low radioiodine uptake in a thyrotoxic female. International Journal of Endocrinology and Metabolism. 2012;**10**:625-628. DOI: 10.5812/ijem.5406

[94] Eskes SA, Endert E, Fliers E, Geskus RB, Dullaart RPF, Links TP, et al. Treatment of amiodarone-induced thyrotoxicosis type 2: A randomized clinical trial. The Journal of Clinical Endocrinology and Metabolism. 2012;**97**:499-506. DOI: 10.1210/jc.2011-2390

[95] Henry RK, Chaudhari M. In iodine-induced thyrotoxicosis, steroid therapy today could keep the surgical knife at bay. Journal of Pediatric Endocrinology & Metabolism. 2018;**31**:585-588. DOI: 10.1515/jpem-2017-0485

Section 3

Nodular Goiter

Chapter 6

Thyroid Nodule: Approach and Management

Madhukar Mittal, Vanishri Ganakumar, Ravindra Shukla and Mahendra Kumar Garg

Abstract

A thyroid nodule is a discrete radiologically distinct lesion in the gland parenchyma. These are a common finding in the general population, majority being diagnosed incidentally during neck imaging. The major clinical relevance lies in the fact that 4–6.5% of nodules can be malignant. A thorough clinical evaluation and examination should be followed by serum TSH assessment and ultrasonography for assessment of size, number, imaging characteristics suggestive of malignancy, cervical lymphadenopathy. FNA should be done based on clinical and sonographic characteristics. Further choice of management modality and extent of surgery should be based on cytopathological findings supplemented by molecular testing if available.

Keywords: thyroid nodule, toxic adenoma, multinodular goitre, thyroiditis

1. Introduction

A thyroid nodule is defined as a discrete radiologically distinct lesion from the surrounding thyroid parenchyma. Nodules which are palpable but do not correspond to distinct abnormalities on ultrasound do not fall under this category [1]. Clinically they can be identified by the doctor on examination or even noticed by the patient themselves. With the increasingly popular use of neck imaging modalities, thyroid nodules are being commonly identified during these imaging studies.

The clinical importance lies in excluding malignancy in a thyroid nodule, assessing functional status, associated with pain at appearance and compressive symptoms (if large) and accordingly decide the line of management. The key guidelines included to cover this area include

1. The 2015 American Thyroid Association Management Guidelines for Adult Patients with Thyroid Nodules and Differentiated Thyroid Cancer.

2. AACE/ACE/AME Task Force on Thyroid Nodules. American Association of Clinical Endocrinologists, American College of Endocrinology, and Associazione Medici Endocrinologi medical guidelines for clinical practice for the diagnosis and management of thyroid nodules-2016 update [2].

3. ACR Thyroid Imaging, Reporting and Data System (TI-RADS): white paper of the ACR TI-RADS Committee [3].

4. European Thyroid Association guidelines for ultrasound malignancy risk stratification of thyroid nodules in adults: The EU-TIRADS [4].

This chapter thus provides a comprehensive coverage of the topic with an optimal approach in management of a thyroid nodule.

2. Epidemiology

Thyroid nodules are a common finding in general population. This is likely due to the increased use of diagnostic imaging for purposes unrelated to the thyroid. The prevalence of thyroid nodules in a population depends on the screening method used and the presence of risk factors for nodule development. The prevalence of thyroid nodules by palpation was found to be 4.2% in a population-based study in Framingham. The prevalence in females and males was 6.4 and 1.5%, respectively [5]. Clinically nonpalpable nodules are frequently identified on ultrasonography and are termed "incidentalomas." The prevalence of thyroid nodules as detected by high resolution ultrasound can be as high as 67% [6]. The prevalence in this Californian study also had an asymmetrical distribution with 72 and 41% prevalence in females and males respectively. 22% patients had solitary nodules, whereas 45% had multiple nodules. In another Italian study by Bartollota et al., the prevalence of thyroid nodules by ultrasonography was 33.1%. Thus it becomes a difficult dilemma on what to do with incidentally detected thyroid nodules which are not malignant and not well-characterised.

Also the number of detected nodules increases with age, with the highest prevalence in the seventh decade. Autopsy studies provide the true prevalence of the incidence in a population. An autopsy study in Mayo clinic revealed a prevalence of around 50% even in patients with no history of thyroid disease [7, 8]. This makes it even more complicated that many individuals would complete their lifespan without any intervention for their thyroid nodules.

3. Risk factors

The prevalence of thyroid nodules is 4 times more common in females than in males. Gender disparity is postulated to occur secondary to influence of oestrogen and progesterone, as demonstrated by increased risk associated with pregnancy and multiparity [9]. The prevalence of thyroid nodules increases with age. Nodules occur more commonly in areas of iodine deficiency. Cigarette smoking can also predispose to development of nodular goitre. This can occur secondary to inhibition of iodine uptake and organification by thiocyanate, which is derived from cyanide in cigarette smoke, hence mimicking iodine deficiency [10]. Obesity has also been demonstrated to be associated with increased risk of goitre and thyroid nodules [11, 12]. Serum IGF-1, being a potent mitogenic factor, was postulated to be associated with development of thyroid nodules. A positive association was observed between serum IGF-1 levels and prevalence of thyroid nodules in males in a study by Volzke et al. In a study by Ying Jian Liu et al., serum IGF-1 levels were not found to be significantly different in patients with hot nodules, cystic cold and solid cold nodules. However, in subgroup analysis, patients with thyroid adenoma on FNA were found to be having significantly higher serum IGF1 levels compared to the control group comprising of healthy adults. However no such association was demonstrated in a study by Hsiao et al. [13–15]. On the other hand, alcohol intake has been associated with decreased prevalence of goitre and thyroid nodules [16].

Autoimmune thyroid diseases are commonly associated with thyroid nodules. Graves disease is associated with nodules in 10–31% of patients. In a Brazilian study, the prevalence of nodules in Graves disease was 27.8%; 19.5% of the nodules harboured thyroid carcinomas, yielding an overall malignancy prevalence of 5% in patients with Graves disease. Younger age and increased thyroid volumes were associated with increased risk for papillary thyroid carcinoma (PTC). This was in contrast to other studies where older age was a risk factor for malignancy [17, 18]. Small thyroid nodules are also commonly associated with Hashimotos thyroiditis. These should be differentiated form pseudonodules resulting from inflammatory infiltrate. Despite the concerns, the US Preventive Services Task Force (USPSTF), which reviews the effectiveness of screening programs in asymptomatic individuals, recommended against screening for thyroid cancer in adults without signs or symptoms of the disease [19].

4. Aetiology

Thyroid nodular disease comprises of a wide range of disorders. Colloid nodules, cysts and thyroiditis comprise of 80% of cases, whereas benign follicular neoplasms and thyroid carcinomas account for 10–15% and 5% cases respectively [20]. These causes have been summarised in **Table 1**.

Benign causes	Malignant causes
Hashimotos thyroiditis	Papillary thyroid carcinoma (PTC)
Colloid adenomas	Follicular thyroid carcinoma (FTC)
Cysts	Medullary thyroid carcinoma (MTC)
Follicular adenomas	Anaplastic thyroid carcinoma (ATC)
Hurthle cell adenomas	Primary thyroid lymphoma
	Metastatic carcinomas (breast, renal, lung, head and neck)

Table 1.
Aetiology of thyroid nodules.

5. Clinical evaluation

Thyroid nodules can present as anterior neck swelling. Most nodules grow very slowly over years. Patients may also present with history of rapid increase in size, which can be suggestive of a malignancy, or a haemorrhage into a nodule, especially if associated with pain. Significant sized nodules can result in compressive symptoms based on the anatomical structure being compromised. Larger nodules can result in compression of underlying structures leading to symptoms like dyspnoea, dysphagia, and hoarseness of voice with compression of trachea, oesophagus and recurrent laryngeal nerves respectively. Patient can also present with thyroid dysfunction. Younger patients with adenoma and thyrotoxicosis (Toxic adenoma) tend to present with the classical symptoms of thyrotoxicosis like nervousness, weight loss despite increased appetite, tremors, palpitations, heat intolerance and sweating. On the other hand, thyrotoxicosis in elderly can present with non-specific symptoms like anorexia, atrial fibrillation, congestive heart failure, and is difficult to diagnose due to lack of classical symptoms. A hypothyroid presentation with fatigue, constipation, cold intolerance is more indicative of a diagnosis of autoimmune thyroiditis in patients with nodular goitre.

History	Findings
Age < 20 years or > 70 years	Nodules >4 cm in size
Male sex	Hard consistency
Increasing size/rapid growth	Fixed nodule
Compressive symptoms: dyspnoea, dysphagia, hoarseness of voice	Vocal cord palsy
Childhood H/O exposure to radiation	Regional lymphadenopathy
Family H/O thyroid malignancies, MEN2, intestinal polyposis syndromes	Distant metastases

Table 2.
Risk factors for malignancy.

Findings suggestive of hyperthyroidism or hypothyroidism should be actively elicited during examination. Size of the gland and qualitative and quantitative description of palpable nodules and lymph nodes should be noted, including size, tenderness, consistency and fixity to surrounding anatomical structures. Smaller thyroid nodules <1 cm, and posteriorly or substernally located nodules can be difficult to palpate, and would be better characterised by imaging techniques.

Increasingly nodules are being detected during neck imaging for other indications. The clinical importance of diagnosis of thyroid nodules lies in excluding malignancy in these patients. 4–6.5% of thyroid nodules can harbour malignancy [1]. History of rapid growth of the nodule, hoarseness of voice due to paralysis of vocal cords suggests a malignant aetiology. Examination features in such cases could include a hard consistency of the nodule, fixation to surrounding structures, presence of regional lymphadenopathy or distant metastases. The risk of a nodule being malignant increases with extremes of age and with male sex. The frequency of malignancy in patients with solitary nodules is not different from nodules seen in multinodular thyroid disease [21].

Other risk factors which impart increased risk of malignancy should be enquired in all patients. History of prior exposure to radiation for various indications like haematopoietic malignancies and stem cell transplantation, head and neck, mediastinal and CNS tumours should be sought, as this increases the likelihood of malignancy in thyroid nodules. Familial forms of thyroid cancers should be considered in differential diagnosis in the presence of supportive history. Most common form of familial thyroid cancers is seen in medullary thyroid carcinomas (MTC). Familial MTC can occur either as an isolated problem inherited in an autosomal dominant fashion, or as a component of MEN 2A (MTC, primary hyperparathyroidism, pheochromocytoma) MEN 2B (MTC, pheochromocytoma, ganglioneuromas, Marfanoid habitus, thickened corneal nerves). Familial papillary thyroid carcinoma (PTC) can occur as an autosomally dominantly inherited isolated form, or can be a component of Pendred syndrome or intestinal polyposis syndromes like Familial adenomatous polyposis (FAP), Gardner syndrome and Peutz Jeghers syndrome. Follicular thyroid carcinoma (FTC) can be associated with Cowden disease and Bannayan Riley Ruvalcaba syndrome. Carney complex type I can be associated with either PTC or FTC, whereas Werner's syndrome can be associated with PTC, FTC or anaplastic thyroid carcinoma (ATC) [22]. Factors suggestive of an increased likelihood of malignancy have been summarised in **Table 2**.

6. Laboratory evaluation

6.1 Serum TSH

The initial evaluation in all patients presenting with a thyroid nodule should include a measurement of serum TSH. If TSH levels are low, possibility of subclinical or overt hyperthyroidism should be considered. Approximately 10% of solitary nodules can be associated with a subnormal TSH. Multinodular goitres, on the other hand, are frequently associated with suppressed TSH due to development of autonomy in the nodules. Serum free T4 levels and T3 levels should be obtained for documentation of hyperthyroidism; the latter may especially be obtained in areas with iodine deficiency due to preferential secretion of T3 over T4 in these circumstances. Patients with a thyroid nodule and subnormal TSH can be taken for a Nuclear Thyroid Scan to document the functional status of the nodule.

6.2 Serum thyroid antibodies

In patients with elevated TSH, anti-thyroid peroxidase (anti-TPO) antibodies may be measured which point to a diagnosis of Hashimotos thyroiditis. However, positive anti-TPO does not obviate the need for a cytopathological evaluation, as a coexisting malignancy needs to be ruled out. A raised or even a normal TSH is associated with an increased risk of malignancy, as well as a more advanced stage of differentiated thyroid cancer [23, 24].

6.3 Serum thyroglobulin

Thyroglobulin (Tg) is a storage form of thyroid hormones, synthesised by thyroid follicular cells. Serum Tg levels are elevated in many benign and malignant thyroid disorders. An elevated level of serum Tg cannot differentiate malignancy in a thyroid nodule with certainty. Measurement of serum thyroglobulin has a role in postoperative monitoring for residual, recurrent or metastatic disease in patients with differentiated thyroid cancers.

6.4 Serum calcitonin

Calcitonin is produced by the parafollicular C cells of the thyroid gland and is a marker for medullary thyroid cancer (MTC). Basal and pentagastrin stimulated serum calcitonin has a role in early diagnosis as well as post-operative monitoring of patients with MTC. Serum calcitonin is measured in patients with family history of MTC or MEN-2 syndrome. Unstimulated serum calcitonin levels >50–100 pg/ml are commonly associated with MTC. There are no recommendations for the routine use of calcitonin in evaluation of thyroid nodules in current recommendations.

7. Imaging

7.1 Radionuclide scan

Hyper-functioning thyroid nodules comprise up to 10% of thyroid nodules. Currently ATA recommends performing a thyroid radionuclide scan in patients with thyroid nodule associated with subnormal TSH. Two radionuclides are primarily used for functional evaluation of thyroid nodules: I123 and Tc 99 m pertechnetate. Both the radioisotopes are taken up by thyroid follicular cells, but only radioiodine is organified and stored within the gland. A thyroid nodule can be classified as "hot/hyperfunctioning", "warm/isofunctioning" and "cold/hypo-functioning" on scintigraphy. A functioning nodule is nearly always benign. 5% of nodules that appear hot or warm on pertechnetate scanning can appear cold on radioiodine scanning, up to 30% of which can be malignant [25].

On the contrary, the risk of malignancy in non-functioning nodules is 4–6.5% [26–29]. Since malignancy is rarely encountered in hyperfunctioning nodules, further cytological evaluation is not necessary if a corresponding hot nodule is identified on scintigraphy.

7.2 Ultrasonography

Ultrasonography has become an indispensable tool for the evaluation of thyroid nodules. Ultrasound is easily available, non-invasive and invaluable for dileniation and prognostication in these patients. Ultrasound in the hands of an experienced sonologist enables accurate identification of size, number of nodules, composition, echogenicity, margins, presence and type of calcifications, shape if taller than wide, vascularity and status of cervical lymph nodes. The pattern of sonographic characteristics of a nodule confers a risk for malignancy. Categories of high suspicion nodules are then subjected to invasive modalities like Fine Needle Aspiration (FNA) and cytological evaluation is done. Features with the highest specificities (median > 90%) are microcalcifications, irregular margins and tall shape, even though the sensitivities are significantly low for any single feature.

Ultrasound is also invaluable in assessing the risk of malignancy in lymph nodes. Location of the lymph nodes adds to the diagnosis. Malignant nodes are more likely to occur in levels III, IV and VI than in level II. PTC tumours arising in upper pole of the thyroid may be an exception as they have a propensity to demonstrate skip metastases to levels III and II. Size of >1 cm, ratio of long axis to short axis (also called as Solbiati index of <2), punctate calcification, presence of hyperechogenicity/mixed echogenicity/cystic changes, loss of hilum and peripheral hypervascularity are some of the features predictive of malignancy. While peripheral vascularity has the highest sensitivity of 86%, punctate calcifications are 100% specific for malignant involvement [30, 31]. However, no single sonographic feature is adequately sensitive for determining malignant involvement. Sonographically suspicious lymph nodes ≥8–10 mm in the smallest diameter should therefore undergo FNA to look for evidence of malignant involvement.

Ultrasound Elastography is a novel modality performed with an ultrasound machine using an elastography computational module. It provides a measure of tissue stiffness, and is being used for malignancy risk assessment. In a study by Azizi et al., thyroid nodule stiffness by elastography was an independent predictor of thyroid carcinoma, with a PPV of 36%, comparable to that of microcalcifications. On the contrary, in another study by Moon et al., elastography alone or in combination with grey scale ultrasound showed an inferior performance compared to grey scale ultrasonographic assessment for differentiation of benign and malignant thyroid nodules [32]. Guidelines currently do not recommend universal use or widespread adoption of ultrasound elastography for malignancy risk assessment.

7.3 CT and MRI neck

Since ultrasound is operator dependent and cannot adequately image deep anatomic structures and those acoustically shadowed by bone or air, preoperative cross sectional imaging like CT/MRI can be used as an adjunct in patients with clinical suspicion of advanced disease, like patients with an invasive primary tumour, or clinically apparent multiple or bulky nodal involvement. These modalities permit imaging beyond the routine cervical regions imaged by the ultrasound, like infraclavicular, retropharyngeal, parapharyngeal regions and the mediastinum. These also aid in preoperative planning to accurately delineate the inferior border, extent of laryngeal tracheal, oesophageal or vascular involvement.

Combined ultrasound and CT may have a higher sensitivity for macroscopic nodal metastasis detection preoperatively, compared to ultrasound alone [33, 34].

DOI: http://dx.doi.org/10.5772/intechopen.91627

Contrast enhanced CT helps in the accurate delineation of the primary tumour and the metastatic disease with the surrounding areas. There exists a small risk of precipitating hyperthyroidism due to iodine content in the contrast agents. Iodine from the IV contrast agents is generally cleared within 4–8 weeks of the scan, as assessed by the urinary iodine levels returning to baseline. Hence a waiting period of atleast a month is advisable to allow urinary iodine levels to return to normal before moving forward to the use of diagnostic or therapeutic radioiodine post-operatively. There is no evidence to suggest this could translate into adverse outcome for thyroid cancer patients currently [31, 35]. MRI is prone to respiration artefacts and can be more difficult to interpret by surgeons in the operating room.

7.4 FDG PET

Functional imaging with 18 F – FDG PET is currently not recommended routinely prior to initial surgery. However, it has been widely accepted as a modality for detecting recurrence of differentiated thyroid cancer, particularly in non-iodine avid disease. PET avidity has also been shown to be a strong predictor of poor outcome in metastatic thyroid cancer [31].

7.5 Guidelines for evaluation, reporting and management of thyroid nodules

Sonographic Scoring systems are used to stratify nodules according to risk of malignancy to allow centres for uniform reporting and reduce interobserver variability.

The **American Thyroid Association (ATA)** risk stratifies nodules into high suspicion, intermediate suspicion, low suspicion, very low suspicion and benign categories based on imaging characteristics. The sonographic features have been shown in **Figure 1** and the FNA cut-offs have been summarised in **Table 3**.

Similar to Breast reporting, the **American College of Radiology** has developed a reporting system for thyroid nodules known as **Thyroid Imaging Reporting and Data System (TIRADS)** for risk stratification based on points assigned for

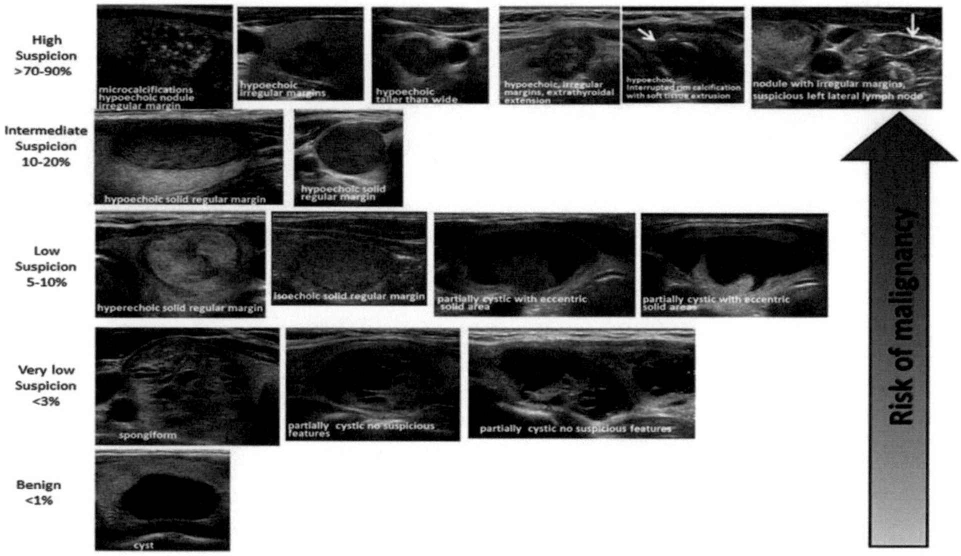

Figure 1.
Sonographic characteristics of thyroid nodules (Adapted from ATA guidelines for adult patients with thyroid nodules and differentiated thyroid cancer [1]).

Sonographic pattern	Ultrasound features	Estimated risk of malignancy	FNA size cutoff (largest dimension)
High suspicion	Solid hypoechoic nodule or solid hypoechoic component of a partially cystic nodule with one or more of the following • Irregular margins (infiltrative, microlobulated) • Microcalcifications • Taller than wider shape • Rim calcifications with small extrusive soft tissue component • Evidence of extrathyroidal extension (ETE)	>70–90%	≥1 cm
Intermediate suspicion	Hypoechoic solid nodule with smooth margins, without microcalcifications, ETE, or taller than wider shape	10–20%	≥1 cm
Low suspicion	Isoechoic or hyperechoic solid nodule, or partially cystic nodule with eccentric solid areas, without microcalcification, irregular margin or ETE or taller than wider shape	5–10%	≥1.5 cm
Very low suspicion	Spongiform or partially cystic nodules without any of the sonographic features described as low, intermediate or high suspicion patterns	<3	≥2 cm/ Observe

Table 3.
Sonographic characteristics and FNA cutoffs of thyroid nodules Adapted from ATA guidelines for adult patients with thyroid nodules and differentiated thyroid cancer [1].

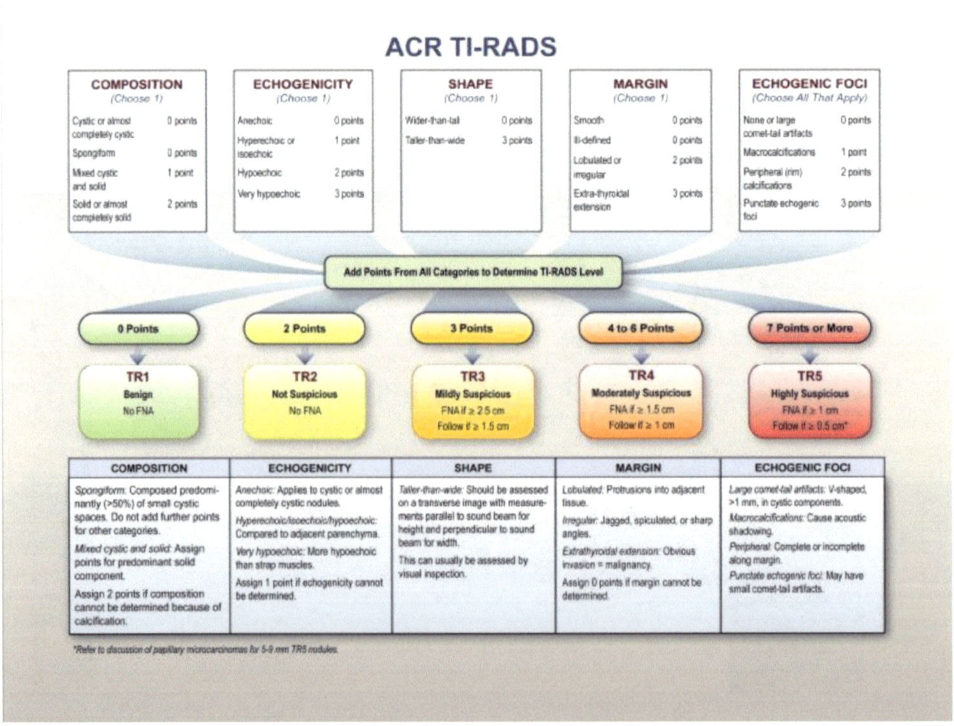

Figure 2.
The ACR-TIRADS scoring system of reporting for thyroid nodules (reproduced from www.acr.org).

composition, echogenicity, shape, margin and echogenic foci in the nodule. The total number of points is then used to classify a nodule into benign (TR1), not suspicious (TR2), mildly suspicious (TR3), moderately suspicious (TR4), and highly suspicious (TR5) categories. This system was proposed in a study by Horvath et al., and the probability of malignancy was 0, 3.4%, 14% and 87% in categories 2, 3, 4 and 5 respectively [36]. FNA is not indicated in TR1 and TR2 categories, whereas FNAC is advised if nodule size is ≥2.5, ≥1.5 and ≥ 1 cm, respectively, in TR3, TR4 and TR5 categories, respectively. The details of the scoring system are shown in **Figure 2**.

Patients with multiple thyroid nodules ≥1 cm should be evaluated similarly as delineated above for patients with solitary nodule. Each nodule in a multinodular gland carries an independent risk of malignancy, and FNA should be done in sequentially based on imaging characteristics. In case of multiple sonologically similar low or very low risk pattern nodules, aspiration can be done in the largest nodule ≥2 cm, or surveillance can be continued without FNA.

8. Fine needle aspiration (FNA)

FNA is the single most valuable, cost effective and accurate method in the evaluation of a nodular goitre. It has demonstrated a sensitivity and specificity of 65–98 and 72–100%, respectively [22]. The use of FNA results in fewer surgeries, reduced cost of care, while improving the malignancy yield at thyroidectomy [37]. Selection of which nodule to subject to FNA is crucial for optimum yield of the procedure. This is based on the sonographic criteria and the size cut-offs depending on which guideline one follows.

FNA is done as an outpatient procedure under local anaesthesia or no anaesthesia. 23–27 guage needles are used to obtain samples for cytopathology. For nodules with a high likelihood of non-diagnostic cytology (>25–50% cystic component) or sampling error (difficult to palpate or posteriorly located), ultrasound guided FNA is preferred [29].

To address variability in reporting thyroid cytopathology, **Bethesda System for reporting thyroid cytopathology** was introduced in 2007. Cytologic adequacy for reporting was defined as presence of at least six groups of well visualised follicular cells, each group containing at least 10 well preserved epithelial cells, preferably on a single slide. The Bethesda system recognises six diagnostic categories and provides an estimation of cancer risk within each category, which has been summarised in **Table 4**.

Diagnostic category	Estimated risk of malignancy by Bethesda system, %	Actual risk of malignancy in surgically excised nodules, % median (range)
Non diagnostic or unsatisfactory	1–4	20 (9–32)
Benign	0–3	2.5 (1–10)
Atypia of undetermined significance or follicular lesion of undetermined significance (AUS/FLUS)	5–15	14 (6–48)
Follicular neoplasm or suspicious for a follicular neoplasm (FN/SFN)	15–30	25 (14–34)
Suspicious for malignancy	60–75	70 (53–97)
Malignant	97–99	99 (94–100)

Table 4.
The Bethesda system for reporting cytopathology: diagnostic categories and risk of malignancy [38].

PTC, MTC and ATC can be diagnosed by cytopathology preoperatively. However, cytopathology cannot differentiate between FTC and follicular adenoma as histopathological findings of vascular and capsular invasion distinguish these entities.

9. Markers and molecular testing

FNA specimens can also be investigated for molecular markers, mutations and rearrangements to assess the risk of malignancy, prognosis and decide further management strategies in cases of indeterminate cytology.

Thyroglobulin and calcitonin in the washout fluid from FNA of cervical lymph nodes can serve as potential markers for metastatic well differentiated thyroid carcinoma and MTC respectively. TG levels of <1 ng/ml in the washout fluid is reassuring, with higher levels corresponding to increasing probability of N1 disease. This is particularly useful in cases in which lymph nodes are cystic, cases with inadequate cytological evaluation and sono-cytological discordance [1].

The 2 most common molecular testing strategies are **mutational analysis** and **gene expression analysis (GEC)**, in which genetic information can be derived from the sample obtained in the original fine-needle aspiration.

Mutational analysis involves isolating DNA from thyroid follicular cells in the specimen and performing gene sequencing. For example, RET-PTC and AKAP9/BRAF rearrangements, BRAF mutations can be associated with PTC and ATC of PTC origin. PTCs with BRAF mutation tend to be more aggressive, with greater propensity for extrathyroidal invasion and a more advanced clinical stage. FTCs are commonly associated with PAX8/PPARγ fusion in 20–50% of cases, followed by RAS mutations. The presence of markers like calcitonin and RET protein are suggestive of MTC. RET mutations are associated with fMTC, MEN2A and MEN 2B [22]. The seven gene mutation and rearrangement panel comprising of BRAF, NRAS, HRAS and KRAS point mutations, and rearrangements of RET/PTC1 and 3, and PAX8/PPARγ has a high specificity of 86–100% and a PPV of 84–100%, but poor sensitivity of 44–100%. It is being used as a **rule in test** for thyroid malignancy. However, while mutations in *RAS* genes (*HRAS*, *KRAS*, *NRAS*) are present in thyroid cancers, they are also present in nonmalignant thyroid neoplasms and in noninvasive follicular thyroid neoplasm with papillary-like nuclear features (NIFTP), and are therefore less specific. Furthermore, if no mutations are found, a thyroid malignancy with a mutation that was not assessed could still be present (~4%); therefore, mutational testing may lead to both false-negative and false-positive results, especially if *RAS* mutations are found.

The second type of molecular testing, gene expression classifier (GEC), uses a proprietary algorithm to analyse the expression of specific genes, the Afirma gene expression classifier (167 GEC), i.e. the mRNA expression of 167 genes, evaluates for the presence of a benign gene expression profile, with a high sensitivity of 92% and NPV of 93%, but low PPV and specificity of 48–53%. Hence it is used as a **rule out test** to identify benign nodules that do not require surgery. However one needs to bear in mind that nodules with a benign GEC result still have a 5% risk of malignancy [28]. MicroRNA analysis is a more recent method for molecular testing for which limited data is available.

10. Management

10.1 Toxic adenoma and toxic multinodular goitre

Patients with toxic adenoma and toxic multinodular goitre (Toxic MNG) can be managed with either radioactive iodine ablation (RAIA) or surgery with surgery being preferred for Toxic MNG and RAIA for Toxic adenoma. For patients with toxic adenoma, the risk of treatment failure is <1% after surgical resection (ipsilateral thyroid lobectomy or isthmusectomy), whereas the risk of persistent hyperthyroidism and recurrent hyperthyroidism with radioiodine therapy is 6–18 and 3–5.5%, respectively. For patients with toxic multinodular goitre, the risk of treatment failure is <1% following surgery (near-total/total thyroidectomy), compared with 20% risk of need for retreatment following radioiodine therapy.

Radioiodine therapy may additionally be preferred in the following scenarios:

- Advanced patient age
- Comorbidities with increased surgical risk
- Small goitre size
- RAIU sufficient to allow therapy
- Previously operated or irradiated necks
- Lack of access to a high volume thyroid surgeon

Radioiodine therapy is contraindicated in pregnancy, lactation, coexisting thyroid cancer, inability to comply with radiation safety guidelines.

Surgery (near total/total thyroidectomy for multinodular goitre, ipsilateral thyroid lobectomy or isthmusectomy for toxic adenoma) can be preferred in the following scenarios:

- Symptomatic compression or large goitres >80 g
- Need for rapid correction of the thyrotoxic state
- Substernal or retrosternal extension
- Relatively low uptake of RAI
- Documented or suspected thyroid malignancy
- Large thyroid nodules, especially if >4 cm
- Coexisting hyperparathyroidism requiring surgery

In patients who are poor candidates for either therapies, long term anti-thyroid drugs (ATDs) can be considered as an alternative [39].

10.2 Management of thyroid nodule based on FNA findings

If a nodule is found benign on cytology, no further immediate diagnostic studies or treatment is required. Infact more than 90% of detected thyroid nodules need no intervention because they have no ultrasound features to suggest malignancy or because they are cytologically benign.

Nodules with high suspicion pattern on ultrasound can be followed up with a repeat ultrasound and FNA within 12 months, whereas nodules with low to intermediate suspicion can have a repeat ultrasound at 12–24 months. If sonographic evidence of growth (>20% increase in atleast two nodule dimensions, with a minimal increase of 2 mm, increase in volume by 50%) or appearance of a suspicious sonographic pattern, FNA should be repeated or monitoring continued with repeat ultrasound, with repeat FNA in case of continued growth. Nodules with very low suspicion pattern can have a repeat ultrasound at ≥24 months if >1 cm, rest do not require a routine sonographic follow up. If a nodule has a second benign cytology on repeat ultrasound guided FNA, then further surveillance with ultrasound is not required. Surgery may be considered in growing nodules >4 cm, presence of compressive symptoms or cosmetic concern. There is no role of levothyroxine suppression therapy in benign thyroid nodules.

For nodules with AUS/FLUS cytology, repeat FNA and molecular testing may be used to supplement malignancy risk assessment in addition to clinical and sonographic features. Mutational testing for BRAF in AUS/FLUS samples has high specificity, but low sensitivity for cancer. Testing for the seven gene panel of mutations and rearrangements (BRAF, NRAS, KRAS, HRAS, RET/PTC1, RET/PTC3, PAX8/PPARγ) offer a significantly higher sensitivity of 63–80%. On the other hand, molecular testing using the 167 GEC (gene expression classifier) in AUS/FLUS cytology has yielded a sensitivity and NPV of 90 and 95%, respectively, but only 53% specificity and 38% PPV for cancer. If repeat FNA and molecular testing are not performed or both are inconclusive, either surveillance or diagnostic surgical excision may be carried out based on clinical and sonographic risk factors and patient preference.

If cytology is suggestive of FN/SFN, diagnostic surgical excision is the long-established standard of care. Clinical, sonographic pattern and molecular testing may be used to supplement the malignancy risk assessment. Testing for the seven gene panel of mutations in FN/SFN cytology has a sensitivity of 57–75%, specificity of 97–100%, PPV of 87–100%, NPV of 79–86%. Molecular testing with GEC is reported to have a 94% NPV, and a 37% PPV in the FN/SFN subgroup. If molecular testing is unavailable, a diagnostic surgical excision is the preferred treatment modality. No further treatment is required if the histopathology of surgical specimen is suggestive of a follicular adenoma. However, if the histopathology is suggestive of FTC, then a completion thyroidectomy may be required.

If the cytology is suspicious of papillary carcinoma (SUSP), surgical management is similar to that of malignant cytology, depending on clinical risk factors, sonographic characteristics and mutational testing if available. BRAF testing is estimated to have 36% sensitivity and 100% specificity, whereas testing with seven gene panel is reported to have 50–68% sensitivity, 86–96% specificity, 80–95% PPV and 70–75% NPV in this subgroup. On the other hand, GEC testing has a PPV (76%) similar to cytology, and a NPV of 85%, hence is not indicated in this cytological diagnosis. Molecular testing may be done if expected to alter the surgical decision making.

For a nodule with initial non diagnostic cytology, repeat FNA should be done with ultrasound guidance, and with on-site cytological evaluation if available. If the results are repeatedly non diagnostic, surgery should be considered for histopathological diagnosis in the presence of clinical and sonographic risk factors for malignancy, or growth of the nodule >20% in two dimensions detected during ultrasound surveillance.

Surgical management in cytologically indeterminate nodules (AUS/FLUS, FN/SFN, SUSP) can be either hemithyroidectomy or near total or total thyroidectomy based on clinical risk factors (nodule >4 cm, family history, history of radiation) and findings on sonography, cytology and molecular testing.

If cytology is diagnostic of a primary thyroid malignancy, then thyroid surgery is the treatment of choice. The choice of surgery depends on the stage of the differentiated thyroid cancer. In tumours ≥4 cm, or with gross extrathyroidal invasion or clinically apparent nodal metastasis or distant metastasis, near total or total thyroidectomy is the treatment of choice. Therapeutic central compartment neck dissection should accompany the procedure in case of clinical involvement of central nodes. Therapeutic lateral neck compartmental neck dissection should be undertaken in case of biopsy proven metastatic lateral cervical lymphadenopathy. Prophylactic central compartment neck dissection can be considered in cases of papillary thyroid carcinoma with advanced primary tumour (T3/T4), or clinically involved lateral neck nodes.

For thyroid cancers >1 cm and < 4 cm, with no gross extrathyroidal invasion/ nodal or distant metastasis, either lobectomy or near-total/total thyroidectomy can be considered. In tumours <1 cm, without extrathyroidal extension and nodal involvement, the initial surgical procedure should be a lobectomy, unless there are clear indications to remove the contralateral lobe. Active surveillance can be chosen in very low risk tumours like micropapillary carcinoma (tumour ≤1 cm), patients at high surgical risk or limited life expectancy [1].

Newer minimally invasive methods like percutaneous ethanol ablation, radiofrequency, laser, microwave ablation, and high-intensity focused ultrasound have been tried and may be considered for treating clinically relevant benign thyroid nodules [40]. Recurrent cystic thyroid nodules with benign cytology can be considered for percutaneous ethanol injection (PEI) or surgical excision. Ethanol acts by coagulative necrosis and small vessel thrombosis.

10.3 Management in specific situations: pregnancy

Thyroid nodules may enlarge slightly during pregnancy, though this does not imply malignant transformation. Patients with suppressed TSH beyond 16 weeks of pregnancy should be monitored until after delivery and cessation of lactation, followed by a radionuclide scan to assess the functional status of the nodule if TSH is still suppressed.

In euthyroid and hypothyroid patients, FNA should be done if clinically and sonographically indicated similar to non-pregnant patients. If PTC is diagnosed by cytology during pregnancy, surgery should be considered during pregnancy only if there is substantial growth (>20% increase in atleast two nodule dimensions, with a minimal increase of 2 mm, increase in volume by 50%) before 24–26 weeks of gestation, or if ultrasound reveals cervical nodes suspicious of metastatic disease. The surgery should be carried out in second trimester before 24 weeks to minimise the risk of miscarriage. If the disease remains stable by mid gestation, or diagnosed in second half of the pregnancy, surgery may be deferred until after delivery. As higher TSH levels may correlate with a more advanced stage of cancer, thyroid hormone therapy can be initiated if TSH > 2 mIU/L, with a target TSH of 0.3–2 mIU/L for the remainder of gestation.

11. Conclusion

Thyroid nodules pose a common clinical problem to physicians and surgeons alike. The primary concern in the evaluation of thyroid nodules is exclusion of malignancy while bearing in mind that most thyroid nodules are benign. With the advent and easy availability of high-resolution ultrasound, reliable of characterisation is possible while deciding on further testing for FNA. FNA is the single most valuable cost effective and reliable investigation for risk stratification, complemented by clinical risk factors. New molecular markers can aid in risk stratification in nodules with indeterminate cytology. Diagnostic surgical excision can be done in these patients if associated with high risk clinical and sonographic features. Patients with malignant cytology should undergo surgery. Evidence based practices should be followed while keeping in mind patient preferences thus giving individualized precision medical care for patients with thyroid nodule.

Author details

Madhukar Mittal*, Vanishri Ganakumar, Ravindra Shukla and
Mahendra Kumar Garg
Department of Endocrinology, All India Institute of Medical Sciences, Jodhpur, India

*Address all correspondence to: mittalspace@gmail.com

References

[1] Haugen BR, Alexander EK, Bible KC, Doherty GM, Mandel SJ, Nikiforov YE, et al. 2015 American Thyroid Association management guidelines for adult patients with thyroid nodules and differentiated thyroid cancer: The American Thyroid Association guidelines task force on thyroid nodules and differentiated thyroid cancer. Thyroid. 2016;**26**(1):1-133

[2] Gharib H, Papini E, Garber JR, et al. AACE/ACE/AME task force on thyroid nodules. American Association of Clinical Endocrinologists, American College of Endocrinology, and Associazione Medici Endocrinologi medical guidelines for clinical practice for the diagnosis and management of thyroid nodules-2016 update. Endocrine Practice. 2016;**22**(5):622-639

[3] Tessler FN, Middleton WD, Grant EG, et al. ACR thyroid imaging, reporting and data system (TI-RADS): White paper of the ACR TI-RADS Committee. Journal of the American College of Radiology. 2017;**14**(5):587-595

[4] Russ G, Bonnema SJ, Erdogan MF, Durante C, Ngu R, Leenhardt L. European thyroid association guidelines for ultrasound malignancy risk stratification of thyroid nodules in adults: The EU-TIRADS. European Thyroid Journal. 2017;**6**(5):225-237

[5] Vander JB, Gaston EA, Dawber TR. The significance of nontoxic thyroid nodules. Final report of a 15-year study of the incidence of thyroid malignancy. Annals of Internal Medicine. 1968; **69**(3):537-540

[6] Bartolotta TV, Midiri M, Runza G, Galia M, Taibbi A, Damiani L, et al. Incidentally discovered thyroid nodules: Incidence, and greyscale and colour Doppler pattern in an adult population screened by real-time compound spatial sonography. La Radiologia Medica. 2006;**111**(7):989-998

[7] Dean DS, Gharib H. Epidemiology of thyroid nodules. Best Practice & Research. Clinical Endocrinology & Metabolism. 2008;**22**(6):901-911

[8] Mortensen JD, Woolner LB, Bennett WA. Gross and microscopic findings in clinically normal thyroid glands. The Journal of Clinical Endocrinology and Metabolism. 1955;**15**(10):1270-1280

[9] Popoveniuc G, Jonklaas J. Thyroid nodules. The Medical Clinics of North America. 2012;**96**(2):329-349

[10] Lio S, Napolitano G, Marinuzzi G, Monaco F. Role of smoking in goiter morphology and thyrotropin response to TRH in untreated goitrous women. Journal of Endocrinological Investigation. 1989;**12**(2):93-97

[11] Wang N, Fang H, Fu C, Huang P, Su M, Jiang F, et al. Associations of adiposity measurements with thyroid nodules in Chinese children living in iodine-sufficient areas: An observational study. BMJ Open. 1 October 2017;**7**(10):e016706

[12] de Sousa PAM, Vaisman M, Carneiro JRI, Guimarães L, Freitas H, Pinheiro MFC, et al. Prevalence of goiter and thyroid nodular disease in patients with class III obesity. Arquivos Brasileiros de Endocrinologia e Metabologia. 2013;**57**(2):120-125

[13] Völzke H, Friedrich N, Schipf S, Haring R, Lüdemann J, Nauck M, et al. Association between serum insulin-like growth factor-I levels and thyroid disorders in a population-based study. The Journal of Clinical Endocrinology and Metabolism. 2007;**92**(10):4039-4045

[14] Hsiao PJ, Tsai JH. Increased insulin-like growth factor-1 receptors in thyroid tissues of graves' disease. Journal of

the Formosan Medical Association. 1994;**93**(11-12):925-932

[15] Liu Y-J, Qiang W, Liu X-J, Xu L, Guo H, Wu L-P, et al. Association of insulin-like growth factor-1 with thyroid nodules. Oncology Letters. Nov 2011;**2**(6):1297-1301

[16] Risk Factors for Goiter and Thyroid Nodules|Thyroid [Internet]. 2019. Available from: https://www.liebertpub.com/doi/pdf/10.1089/105072502761016502

[17] Senyurek Giles Y, Fatih T, Harika B, Yersu K, Tarik T, Serdar T. The risk factors for malignancy in surgically treated patients for graves' disease, toxic multinodular goiter, and toxic adenoma. Surgery. 2008;**144**(6):1028-1037

[18] Kim WB, Han S-M, Kim TY, Nam-Goong IS, Gong G, Lee HK, et al. Ultrasonographic screening for detection of thyroid cancer in patients with graves' disease. Clinical Endocrinology. 2004;**60**(6):719-725

[19] Bibbins-Domingo K, Grossman DC, Curry SJ, Barry MJ, Davidson KW, Doubeni CA, et al. Screening for thyroid cancer: US preventive services task force recommendation statement. Journal of the American Medical Association. 2017;**317**(18):1882-1887

[20] Hegedüs L. Clinical practice. The thyroid nodule. The New England Journal of Medicine. 2004;**351**(17):1764-1771

[21] Belfiore A, La Rosa GL, La Porta GA, Giuffrida D, Milazzo G, Lupo L, et al. Cancer risk in patients with cold thyroid nodules: Relevance of iodine intake, sex, age, and multinodularity. The American Journal of Medicine. 1992;**93**(4):363-369

[22] Niedziela M. Thyroid nodules. Best Practice & Research. Clinical Endocrinology & Metabolism. 2014;**28**(2):245-277

[23] Haymart MR, Repplinger DJ, Leverson GE, Elson DF, Sippel RS, Jaume JC, et al. Higher serum thyroid stimulating hormone level in thyroid nodule patients is associated with greater risks of differentiated thyroid cancer and advanced tumor stage. The Journal of Clinical Endocrinology and Metabolism. 2008;**93**(3):809-814

[24] Golbert L, de Cristo AP, Faccin CS, Farenzena M, Folgierini H, Graudenz MS, et al. Serum TSH levels as a predictor of malignancy in thyroid nodules: A prospective study. PLoS One. 2017;**12**(11):e0188123

[25] Reschini E, Ferrari C, Castellani M, Matheoud R, Paracchi A, Marotta G, et al. The trapping-only nodules of the thyroid gland: Prevalence study. Thyroid. 2006;**16**(8):757-762

[26] Werk EE, Vernon BM, Gonzalez JJ, Ungaro PC, McCoy RC. Cancer in thyroid nodules. A community hospital survey. Archives of Internal Medicine. 1984;**144**(3):474-476

[27] Belfiore A, Giuffrida D, La Rosa GL, Ippolito O, Russo G, Fiumara A, et al. High frequency of cancer in cold thyroid nodules occurring at young age. Acta Endocrinologica. 1989;**121**(2):197-202

[28] Lin J-D, Chao T-C, Huang B-Y, Chen S-T, Chang H-Y, Hsueh C. Thyroid cancer in the thyroid nodules evaluated by ultrasonography and fine-needle aspiration cytology. Thyroid. 2005;**15**(7):708-717

[29] Tamhane S, Gharib H. Thyroid nodule update on diagnosis and management. Clinical Diabetes and Endocrinology. 1 December 2016;**2**(1):17

[30] Leboulleux S, Girard E, Rose M, Travagli JP, Sabbah N, Caillou B, et al. Ultrasound criteria of malignancy

for cervical lymph nodes in patients followed up for differentiated thyroid cancer. The Journal of Clinical Endocrinology and Metabolism. 2007;**92**(9):3590-3594

[31] Yeh MW, Bauer AJ, Bernet VA, Ferris RL, Loevner LA, Mandel SJ, et al. American Thyroid Association statement on preoperative imaging for thyroid cancer surgery. Thyroid. 2015;**25**(1):3-14

[32] Moon HJ, Sung JM, Kim E-K, Yoon JH, Youk JH, Kwak JY. Diagnostic performance of gray-scale US and elastography in solid thyroid nodules. Radiology. 2012;**262**(3):1002-1013

[33] Lesnik D, Cunnane ME, Zurakowski D, Acar GO, Ecevit C, Mace A, et al. Papillary thyroid carcinoma nodal surgery directed by a preoperative radiographic map utilizing CT scan and ultrasound in all primary and reoperative patients. Head & Neck. 2014;**36**(2):191-202

[34] Suh CH, Baek JH, Choi YJ, Lee JH. Performance of CT in the preoperative diagnosis of cervical lymph node metastasis in patients with papillary thyroid cancer: A systematic review and meta-analysis. AJNR. American Journal of Neuroradiology. 2017;**38**(1):154-161

[35] Padovani RP, Kasamatsu TS, Nakabashi CCD, Camacho CP, Andreoni DM, Malouf EZ, et al. One month is sufficient for urinary iodine to return to its baseline value after the use of water-soluble iodinated contrast agents in post-thyroidectomy patients requiring radioiodine therapy. Thyroid. 2012;**22**(9):926-930

[36] Horvath E, Majlis S, Rossi R, Franco C, Niedmann JP, Castro A, et al. An ultrasonogram reporting system for thyroid nodules stratifying cancer risk for clinical management. The Journal of Clinical Endocrinology and Metabolism. 2009;**94**(5):1748-1751

[37] Hamberger B, Gharib H, Melton LJ, Goellner JR, Zinsmeister AR. Fine-needle aspiration biopsy of thyroid nodules. Impact on thyroid practice and cost of care. The American Journal of Medicine. 1982;**73**(3):381-384

[38] Cibas ES, Ali SZ. NCI thyroid FNA state of the science conference. The Bethesda system for reporting thyroid cytopathology. American Journal of Clinical Pathology. 2009;**132**(5):658-665

[39] Ross DS, Burch HB, Cooper DS, Greenlee MC, Laurberg P, Maia AL, et al. American Thyroid Association guidelines for diagnosis and management of hyperthyroidism and other causes of thyrotoxicosis. Thyroid. 2016;**26**(10):1343-1421

[40] Papini E, Pacella CM, Misischi I, Guglielmi R, Bizzarri G, Døssing H, et al. The advent of ultrasound-guided ablation techniques in nodular thyroid disease: Towards a patient-tailored approach. Best Practice & Research. Clinical Endocrinology & Metabolism. 2014;**28**(4):601-618

Chapter 7

Multinodular Goiter

Sanjay Saran

Abstract

Multinodular goiter (MNG) is the most common disorder of the thyroid gland. It is highly endemic in iodine-deficient areas; MNG can be seen in almost all individuals with severe iodine-deficient areas. It starts as a diffuse enlargement of the thyroid gland and ends in a nodular enlarged thyroid. Though MNG can be sporadic, there is a strong correlation between occurrence of MNG and iodine deficiency. The characteristic feature of MNG is its functional and structural heterogeneity. The MNG usually presents as neck swelling; rarely it may produce pressure symptoms, i.e., dyspnea, hoarseness of voice, and dysphagia. It can also present with symptoms of hyperthyroidism particularly in long-standing goiter. Imaging particularly ultrasound is very useful to define characteristic of MNG and surrounding structure. The incidence of malignancy in MNG is 4–14%, and risk factors are family history of thyroid carcinoma, history of neck radiation, prior surgery, and presence of cervical lymphadenopathies. Management of MNG can be done by drugs, surgery, and radioiodine (I-131) depending on results of diagnostic evaluation and associated complications.

Keywords: hyperthyroidism, iodine, goiter, MNG, multinodular goiter, thyrotoxicosis

1. Introduction

Goiter is the enlargement of the thyroid gland which can be due to a variety of conditions. Nodular goiter is one of the most common endocrine disorders affecting the thyroid gland. It is endemic to certain populations and regions especially those with iodine deficiency. It also tends to occur with a higher frequency in women and in the fourth to fifth decades of life [1]. The prevalence of goiter is variable worldwide and is correlated with iodine intake of regional populations. In approximately 3600 B.C., Chinese medical writings were the first to show a decrease in size of goiter after ingestion of seaweed and burnt sea sponge, and they continued to remain as effective remedies for goiter worldwide as was documented in the writings of Hippocrates, Galen, Roger, and Arnold [2].

After initiation of iodine prophylaxis programs in over 2100 school girls in the United States in 1917 by David Marine and colleagues, iodized salt was introduced in the United States in 1922 for prevention of endemic goiter. Later in 1930 iodized salt became widely available in the United States [3]. The salt iodization is a good approach for decreasing iodine deficiency in population, as it is a universal foodstuff, inexpensive, and easily available and intake is relatively consistent [4]. Approximately 120 countries, including the UK, Canada, Brazil, China, India, Thailand, and Singapore, have adopted mandatory iodization of all food-grade salt [5]. Currently the WHO recommends daily intake of 150 mcg iodine for adults,

250 mcg for pregnant and lactating women, and 90 mcg for children <2 years of age that can be easily obtained by iodized salt, processed food, and milk products [6]. Prevalence of goiter still remains 4–7% in the United States even after iodine supplementation [7].

Goiter can be classified as solitary or multiple, diffuse or nodular, and toxic or nontoxic on an anatomical and functional basis. The nontoxic goiter is due to abnormalities of iodine supplies or metabolism without any abnormal thyroid function. In children goiter tends to be smaller and diffuse, whereas in older people they are usually large and nodular.

2. Etiology and pathophysiology

Thyroid hormones affect the function of virtually all organ systems of the body; these are critical determinants of brain and somatic development in infants and of metabolic activity in adults. The thyroid gland is regulated to a large extent by the delicate balance between the hypothalamus, pituitary, and thyroid. Thyrotropin-releasing hormones (TRH) are secreted by the hypothalamus which stimulates the secretion of the thyroid-stimulating hormone (TSH), by the pituitary gland. TSH is a major regulator of the thyroid gland which after binding to its receptor on plasma membrane stimulates each and all steps of thyroid hormone synthesis and secretion.

Goiter is an etiologically and pathogenetically complex disease. The specific role of TSH in its pathogenesis has not been unraveled. It has been variously defined and characterized by the increased volume of the thyroid gland with the formation of multiple nodules. Although a number of definitions exist, the most accepted is the thyroid gland weighing over 20–25 g or a volume of over 19 ml in females and 25 ml in males [8].

Grossly, MNG reveals a heterogeneous array of solid/cystic and mixed nodules. Cystic nodules are typically defined as a cystic component >50%. Typically, pathogenesis of MNG thyroid can be attributed to three main processes: diffuse follicular hyperplasia, focal nodular proliferation, and eventual acquisition of functional autonomy. Development of goiter especially in conditions of iodine deficiency or Hashimoto's disease seems to be TSH driven. However, in addition to TSH, several other growth factors, both TSH dependent and independent, have been known to play a role in the pathogenesis of MNG by influencing thyroid follicular cell growth. Chronic stimulation of follicular cells primarily due to TSH leads to follicular hyperplasia, which usually then enters a resting phase leading to the formation of colloid goiter [9]. This long-standing diffuse goiter may develop into MNG with the potential of autonomy in certain nodules. The role of genetic factors especially in nontoxic MNG is not clear, but some role has been suggested by twin studies, family history, female preponderance, etc. [10]. Certain mutations like those affecting the activation of camp cascade (e.g., TSH-r mutations) which stimulates growth and function mutation in genes encoding thyroglobulin (Tg), thyroid peroxidase (TPO), dual oxidase 2 (THOX2), the sodium-iodide symporter gene (SLC5A5), Pendred syndrome gene (SLC26A4), the TSH receptor gene (TSHR gene), the iodotyrosine deiodinase (DEHAL 1), and the thyroid oxidase 2 gene (THOX2) have been found to be responsible in certain cases for the formation of nodules in a patient with MNG [10]. Familial MNGs have been found to be strongly associated with mutations in the miRNA processing gene DICER1 [11]. Environmental factors have also been incriminated in causation of MNG possibly by aggravating the expression of heterogeneity causing the thyroid to grow and perhaps leading to its autonomy. Naturally occurring goitrogens are thought to work by different

Goitrogens	Agent	Action
Millet, soy	Flavonoids	Impairs thyroperoxidase activity
Cassava, sweet potato, sorghum	Cyanogenic glucosides metabolized to thiocyanates	Inhibits iodine thyroidal uptake
Babassu coconut, mandioca	Flavonoids	Inhibits thyroperoxidase
Cruciferous vegetables: cabbage, cauliflower, broccoli, turnips	Glucosinolates	Impairs iodine thyroidal uptake
Seaweed (kelp)	Iodine excess	Inhibits release of thyroidal hormones
Malnutrition	Vitamin A deficiency Iron deficiency	Increases TSH stimulation, Reduces heme-dependent thyroperoxidase thyroidal activity
Selenium	Selenium deficiency	Accumulates peroxides and causes deiodinase deficiency; impairs thyroid hormone synthesis

Adapted and modified from Medeiros-Neto and Knobel [48].

Table 1.
Natural goitrogens associated with goiter prevalence.

mechanisms, leading to impaired thyroid hormone synthesis or thyroid growth (**Table 1**). For example, iodine-rich substances like seaweed and cruciferous and cassava may impair iodine uptake [12]. In addition to this protein energy malnutrition and deficiency of other nutrients like iron and selenium, vitamin a may also be associated with thyroid enlargement if present with iodine-deficient state. The non-functioning nodules in nontoxic MNG may over time evolve into larger autonomous nodules, leading first to a smoldering subclinical hyperthyroid state which may then progress to overt hyperthyroidism [13]. The Marine Lenhart disease is functioning thyroid nodules associated with Graves' disease.

3. Types of goiter

3.1 Toxic MNG

Toxic MNG is a result of activating somatic mutation of the TSH receptor gene that leads to diffuse hyperplasia of thyroid follicular cells independent of TSH regulation [14–16]. MNG with thyrotoxicosis is also known as Plummer's disease. Toxic MNG presented with clinical features similar to other causes of thyrotoxicosis except ophthalmopathy. Incidence of thyrotoxicosis in MNG is related to the duration of the presence of MNG. So it's more common in elderly people who are harboring MNG for a long time. Hormone profile in toxic MNG is seen with suppressed TSH along with normal or elevated thyroid hormones.

3.2 Graves' disease

Graves' disease is an autoimmune disorder caused by anti-TSH receptor antibody. These antibodies interact with TSH receptor and cause increased thyroid hormone synthesis and secretion [17]. Many risk factors have been found in causation of Graves' disease including high iodine intake and stress [18, 19]. Several drugs have also been implicated in etiology of Graves' disease including lithium, interferon α, and alemtuzumab [20–22]. Other autoimmune manifestations associated with Graves' disease are pretibial myxedema and ophthalmopathy. Graves' disease is the most common cause of thyrotoxicosis [23]. It is more common in females and usually presents before 30 years of age. Graves' disease presents with classical symptoms of thyrotoxicosis, i.e., irritability, sleeplessness, palpitations, excessive sweating, heat intolerance, and weight loss.

3.3 Hashitoxicosis

Hashitoxicosis, a term coined from Hashimoto's disease and thyrotoxicosis, is a rare condition seen in patients with autoimmune thyroid disease. Hashitoxicosis presents initially with clinical features of thyrotoxicosis and is associated with high radioiodine uptake similar to Graves' disease [24]. Later on it leads to development of hypothyroidism which is caused by lymphocytic infiltration and autoimmune destruction of thyroid gland similar to Hashimoto's thyroiditis. Anti-TSH receptor antibodies are found in nearly 23% of patients with hashitoxicosis [25].

3.4 Subacute (DeQuervain's) thyroiditis

It is a nonsuppurative thyroiditis caused by viral infection or as a result of post-viral illness. In twin study, some link of genetic association was also found [26]. Subacute thyroiditis is characterized by neck pain and tenderness. Initially disease presents with fever, fatigue, and myalgia along with hyperthyroidism that is followed by euthyroidism and then hypothyroidism, and lastly euthyroidism is achieved. A less or absent uptake is seen by radionuclide uptake study. Color Doppler study reveals low blood flow in the hyperthyroid phase which normalizes once euthyroidism is achieved. On laboratory study TSH remains suppressed, and free T4 and free T3 are raised during the hyperthyroid phase.

3.5 Riedel's thyroiditis

Riedel's thyroiditis is a rare condition of unknown etiology occurring in middle-aged women. In this chronic thyroiditis, thyroid follicles are replaced by fibrous tissue. Association with other autoimmune fibrosclerotic disease, i.e., retroperitoneal fibrosis and sclerosing cholangitis, is also found. Initially patients present with goiter with normal thyroid function but later on become hypothyroid. The diagnosis can be made with FNAC, but sometimes biopsy may be required for confirmation.

4. Clinical evaluation of MNG

MNG is usually detected incidentally during routine examination for evaluation of some other disease. Sometimes the patient seeks help for obvious neck swelling and cosmetic disfigurement of the neck. As MNG becomes palpable once the size is more than 1 centimeter, so large MNG mainly presents with neck swelling. Once MNG is detected, a complete history and physical examination focusing on the thyroid gland and adjacent cervical lymph nodes should be performed. Through history including history of childhood head and neck radiation therapy, total body radiation for bone marrow transplantation, exposure to ionizing radiation from fallout in childhood or adolescence, familial thyroid carcinoma, or thyroid cancer syndrome should be sought [27, 28]. Patients with long-standing MNG are more likely to have clinical features of thyrotoxicosis, and they usually present with subclinical or clinical hyperthyroidism during evaluation. The MNG may present with compressive features, i.e., dyspnea and dysphagia. Respiratory symptoms develop due to tracheal compression. Hoarseness of voice may result from compression of recurrent laryngeal nerve. Very rarely MNG may present with vocal cord palsy, but it is usually seen in malignancy. Retrosternal MNG with thoracic inlet compression can be diagnosed with Pemberton's maneuver, in which raising arm overhead causes flushing and shortness of breath due to compression of neck veins. Information regarding family members, any significant drug use, and radiation exposure should also be enquired. Thyroid examination should be done in sitting position, and during palpation information regarding thyroid shape, nodularity, tenderness, and fixity to the surrounding should be sought. Fixation to trachea, esophagus, and surrounding structure raises the possibility of malignancy. Enlarged painful and tender thyroid can be due to subacute thyroiditis or thyroid abscess. Neck mass with enlarged cervical lymph node again raises suspicion of carcinoma and warrants further evaluation.

5. Laboratory investigation

American Thyroid Association (ATA) recommends serum TSH as the initial laboratory test in evaluation of MNG. If serum TSH is abnormal, then serum FT4 and serum FT3 are recommended to know the thyroid's functioning status. Antithyroid peroxidase (anti TPO) antibody and thyroglobulin (Tg) are other laboratory tests to know about thyroid autoimmunity and Tg gene mutation in patients with MNG. If TSH is high, the risk of malignancy is increased, so it warrants further evaluation with imaging and FNAC [29–30].

6. Imaging study

6.1 Thyroid ultrasonography

Thyroid ultrasound is the most widely accepted imaging modality to know the characteristic of MNG. Ultrasound can give information regarding the number of nodules and the size and location of nodules within the thyroid. It also provides information regarding the presence or absence of any suspicious cervical lymph nodes in the neck. Thyroid sonography can also describe features including composition (solid, cystic proportion, or spongiform), echogenicity, margins, presence and type of calcifications, shape if taller than wide, and vascularity which helps in making decision of FNAC (**Figure 1**). Thyroid ultrasound is commonly used in ultrasound guided FNAC for greater yield in diagnosis.

6.2 Radionuclide scan

Although radionuclide imaging of thyroid gland has been done for a long time, resolution of this modality for thyroid nodule is far behind the ultrasonography [31]. So radionuclide imaging is not having much role in anatomic description of MNG. However radionuclide imaging is very useful in describing physiology of thyroid nodules. If TSH is subnormal, then ATA recommends a radionuclide thyroid scan to know whether nodules are hyperfunctioning ("hot," i.e., tracer uptake is greater than the surrounding normal thyroid), isofunctioning ("warm,"

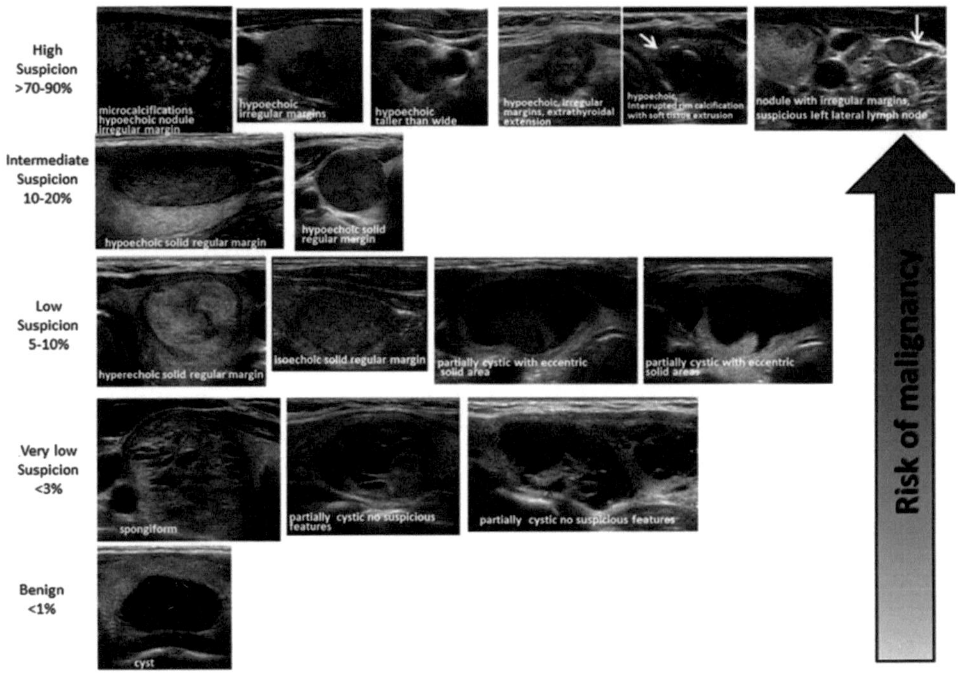

Figure 1.
Nodule sonographic patterns and risk of malignancy.

i.e., tracer uptake is equal to the surrounding thyroid), or nonfunctioning ("cold," i.e., has uptake less than the surrounding thyroid tissue) [32]. Since hyperfunctioning nodules rarely harbor malignancy, so cytologic evaluation is not required in hyperfunctioning nodules. Scan is also useful in distinguishing Graves' disease from (toxic MNG) Plummer's disease.

6.3 CT/MRI

CT/MRI is generally not recommended in evaluation of MNG. These modalities of imaging do not have any advantage over ultrasonography in description of intrathyroidal structure. These imaging modalities are useful only when malignancy is suspected or goiter is retrosternal in which MRI is more precise than CT. CT/MRI provides more information about the surrounding tissue in relation to the thyroid, i.e., trachea, esophagus, and neck vessels. So these imaging modalities are used when features of tracheal compression/deviation, dysphagia, vocal cord paralysis, and weight loss are present. CT/MRI provides additional anatomical information to be helpful preoperatively for planning of surgical excision.

6.4 FNAC

ATA recommends FNAC as the procedure of choice in evaluation of MNG, as it is the cost-effective and most accurate method for thyroid nodule evaluation. FNAC is very reliable and has a low false-negative (7%) and very low false-positive rate near to zero [33]. In one study negative predictive value of case classified as benign was 95% [34]. FNAC provides an algorithm for evaluation and management of patients with thyroid nodules based on sonographic pattern and FNA cytology. ATA recommends FNAC in nodule >1 cm with high or intermediate suspicion of malignancy, nodule >1.5 cm with low suspicion of malignancy, and nodule >2 cm

Diagnostic category	Estimated/predicted risk of malignancy by the Bethesda system, %a	Actual risk of malignancy in nodules surgically excised, % median (range)b
Nondiagnostic or unsatisfactory	1–4	20 (9–32)
Benign	0–3	2.5 (1–10)
Atypia of undetermined significance or follicular lesion of undetermined significance	5–15	14 (6–48)
Follicular neoplasm or suspicious for a follicular neoplasm	15–30	25 (14–34)
Suspicious for malignancy	60–75	70 (53–97)
Malignant	97–99	99 (94–100)

As reported in the Bethesda system by Cibas and Ali.

Table 2.
The Bethesda system for reporting thyroid cytopathology: Diagnostic categories and risk of malignancy.

with very low suspicion of malignancy. FNAC is not recommended for purely cystic nodule. To make a satisfactory FNAC, at least six to eight cell clusters are required in two slides. ATA recommends FNAC to be reported using diagnostic groups outlined in the Bethesda system for reporting thyroid cytopathology (**Table 2**). Based on literature review and expert opinion, the Bethesda system has six diagnostic categories and also provides an estimation of cancer risk within each category. These categories are (i) nondiagnostic/unsatisfactory; (ii) benign; (iii) atypia of undetermined significance/follicular lesion of undetermined significance (AUS/FLUS); (iv) follicular neoplasm/suspicious for follicular neoplasm (FN/SFN), a category that also encompasses the diagnosis of Hu¨rthle cell neoplasm/suspicious for Hürthle cell neoplasm; (v) suspicious for malignancy (susp); and (vi) malignant.

7. Treatment

Treatment of MNG is directed towards existing thyroid disease associated with MNG and etiology of the disease [35]. Management of toxic and nontoxic MNG is done separately and should be based on the type of MNG. Treatment selection is also based on overall health and comorbidities of the patient. Success of treatment depends on the patient selection and type of treatment. Treatment is broadly divided in surgical and nonsurgical modalities. Surgery is indicated in large MNG, retrosternal extension of MNG, compression of trachea or esophagus, rapid growth, suspicion of malignancy, and MNG associated with vocal cord palsy.

7.1 Surgical treatment

Definitive treatment of toxic MNG is done by surgery when goiter size is large. Two types of surgical procedures are performed: total thyroidectomy and subtotal thyroidectomy. In total thyroidectomy all thyroid tissue is surgically excised, whereas in subtotal thyroidectomy small amount of thyroid tissue 1 gm on each lobe of thyroid is left. Before doing surgical procedure, patient should be rendered euthyroid by antithyroid drugs, beta blockers, and potassium iodide or a combination of one or more of these. Preoperatively cardiac evaluation is mandatory, and patient should be stabilized with appropriate treatment. Surgical procedures are the same for toxic and nontoxic MNG. In nontoxic MNG preoperative treatment with antithyroid drugs, beta blockers, or potassium iodide is not required.

Although most surgeons prefer to do total thyroidectomy, still controversy exists regarding the removal of thyroid tissue in between total and subtotal thyroidectomy for surgical treatment of MNG. In study temporary or permanent recurrent laryngeal nerve palsy, temporary or permanent hypoparathyroidism, hemorrhage, and wound complications were not significantly different in total thyroidectomy versus subtotal thyroidectomy [36]. In an analysis, goiter recurrence was significantly more in subtotal thyroidectomy than total thyroidectomy, but reintervention due to goiter was not significantly higher. Incidence of permanent recurrent laryngeal nerve palsy and permanent hypoparathyroidism was more in the total thyroidectomy group, but it was statistically nonsignificant [37]. Postoperatively serum TSH level should be monitored, many physicians prefer to start thyroid hormone as theoretically this may prevent recurrence of goiter, but studies have not shown this kind of benefit from thyroid hormone suppressive therapy [38–39].

7.2 Medical treatment

Levothyroxine (LT4) is used as TSH suppression therapy with variable success for nontoxic goiter. But suppressive therapy with LT4 is associated with thyrotoxicosis particularly in elderly patients. In this subset of patients, it is associated with osteopenia and cardiac arrhythmia and is inversely related to TSH concentration. Very rarely thyroid nodules can become functionally autonomous [40–41]. The goal is to keep TSH in between 0.1 mIU/L and 0.4 mIU/L. However the suppressive therapy is still a matter of debate. A meta-analysis of 11 studies has shown a twofold increase of chance in reduction in nodule size with LT4 suppressive therapy with proper selection of patient [42]. In another study with 54 patients 12 months after starting suppressive therapy, 37.1% of patients with single, solid nodules are found to regress more than 50% in nodule volume, and 20.3% of patients had reduction in nodule volume more than 20% but less than 49.9%. One-third of subjects with MNG had 50% or more regression of the glandular volume, whereas 46.8% were considered as nonresponsive. During suppressive therapy with LT4, the mean serum Tg level was also decreased significantly in these patients [43]. Because of lifelong therapy is required for prevention of goiter recurrence and is associated with risk of autonomous functioning of nodules, so in many patients, TSH suppression with LT4 is not feasible.

Antithyroid drugs propylthiouracil and thionamides (carbimazole and methimazole) are used to restore euthyroidism in toxic MNG. They can be used for a long time in patients whom surgery and radioiodine (I-131) treatment are contraindicated. But risk of agranulocytosis remains a major concern. In a recent study, methimazole was used for 8 years in 53 patients for treatment of toxic MNG without any serious adverse effect [44].

7.3 Radioiodine (I-131)

Radioiodine (I-131) is in use for management of thyroid disorder for more than 50 years. Radioiodine (I-131) is used particularly for thyrotoxic disorder mainly in Graves' disease. Radioiodine (I-131) also causes a significant reduction of thyroid gland volume. Due to its effect on reduction of thyroid gland volume, it has been used in management of nontoxic nodular thyroid disease also. In one study, 35 patients with nontoxic large MNG were treated with mean 1806 mbq (range 800–4000) of I-131. The mean reduction in thyroid volume was 43.18% (range −17.23–89.66%) seen after 3 months of treatment with I-131 [45]. In another study 63.4 ± 3.6% reduction in volume was seen with I-131 in rhTSH-treated nontoxic MNG patients [46]. Treatment with radioiodine (I-131) also relieves symptoms of tracheal and esophagus compression in large MNG. In toxic MNG radioiodine (I-131), euthyroid state is restored in addition to decrease of nodule size in MNG. Pretreatment with rhTSH increases the uptake of radioiodine (I-131) by thyroid tissue in a homogenous manner so that cold areas also take up radioiodine (I-131). In a small study, pretreatment with rhTSH is associated with greater reduction of thyroid volume in radioiodine (I-131)-treated patient [47]. Treatment with radioiodine (I-131) is also associated with adverse effects in a few cases, i.e., hypothyroidism, radiation thyroiditis, and autoimmune hyperthyroidism. Although long-term studies have not demonstrated carcinogenic effect of radioiodine (I-131), still concern regarding thyroid cancer, leukemia, and congenital abnormalities in offspring remains in mind.

8. Conclusion

MNG is the most common thyroid disorder, but usually it is asymptomatic. When large enough it can cause compression to the trachea, esophagus, and neck veins. Other complications of MNG are autonomous functioning nodules, and very rarely it may progress to malignancy. Diagnostic evaluation includes clinical evaluation, thyroid function, and imaging study. Additional testing with FNAC may be required. Treatment modalities include drugs, surgery, and radioiodine (I-131), depending on results of diagnostic evaluation and associated complications.

Author details

Sanjay Saran
Department of Endocrinology, SMS Medical College and Associated Group of Hospitals, Jaipur, Rajasthan, India

*Address all correspondence to: drsanjaysaran@gmail.com

References

[1] Studer H, Gebel F. Sporadic goiter. In: Ingbar SH, Breverman LE, editors. Werner's the Thyroid, a Fundamental and Clinical Text. 5th ed. Philadelphia: LippinCott; 1986. pp. 1311-1315

[2] Rosenfeld L. Discovery and early uses of iodine. Journal of Chemical Education. 2000;**77**:984-987

[3] Dunn JT. What's happening to our iodine? The Journal of Clinical Endocrinology & Metabolism. 1998;**83**:3398-3400

[4] Zimmermann MB. Iodine deficiency and endemic cretinism. In: Braverman LE, Cooper DS, editors. Werner & Ingbar's the Thyroid: A Fundamental and Clinical Text. 10th ed. Philadelphia, PA, USA: Lippincott Williams and Wilkins; 2012. pp. 217-241

[5] Dasgupta PK, Liu Y, Dyke JV. Iodine nutrition: Iodine content of iodized salt in the United States. Environmental Science & Technology. 2008;**42**:1315-1323

[6] WHO Assessment of Iodine Deficiency Disorders and Monitoring Their Elimination: A Guide for Programme Managers; 2018

[7] Daniels GH. Thyroid nodules and nodular thyroids: A clinical overview. Comprehensive Therapy. 1996;**22**:239-250

[8] Teng W, Shan Z, Teng X, Guan H. Effect of iodine intake on thyroid diseases in China. The New England Journal of Medicine. 2006;**354**(26):2783-2793

[9] Taylor S. The evolution of nodular goiter. The Journal of Clinical Endocrinology & Metabolism. 1953;**13**(10):1232-1247

[10] Krohn K, Fuhrer D, Bayer Y, Eszlinger M, Brauer V, Neumann S, et al. Molecular pathogenesis of euthyroid and toxic multinodular goiter. Endocrine Reviews. 2005;**26**(4):504-524

[11] Rio Frio T, Bahubeshi A, Kanellopoulou C, Hamel N, Niedziela M, Sabbaghian N, et al. DICER1 mutations in familial multinodular goiter with and without ovarian Sertoli-Leydig cell tumors. Journal of the American Medical Association. 2011;**305**(1):68-77

[12] Knobel M, Medeiros-Neto G. An outline of inherited disorders of the thyroid hormone generating system. Thyroid. 2003;**13**(8):771-801

[13] Zimmermann MB, Wegmuller R, Zeder C, Chaouki N, Torresani T. The effects of vitamin a deficiency and vitamin a supplementation on thyroid function in goitrous children. The Journal of Clinical Endocrinology & Metabolism. 2004;**89**(11):5441-5447

[14] Duprez L, Hermans J, Van Sande J, et al. Two autonomous nodules of a patient with multinodular goiter harbor different activating mutations of the thyrotropin receptor gene. The Journal of Clinical Endocrinology & Metabolism. 1997;**82**:306

[15] Parma J, Duprez L, Van Sande J, et al. Diversity and prevalence of somatic mutations in the thyrotropin receptor and Gs alpha genes as a cause of toxic thyroid adenomas. The Journal of Clinical Endocrinology & Metabolism. 1997;**82**:2695

[16] Holzapfel HP, Führer D, Wonerow P, et al. Identification of constitutively activating somatic thyrotropin receptor mutations in a subset of toxic multinodular goiters. The Journal of Clinical Endocrinology & Metabolism. 1997;**82**:4229

[17] Davies TF. New thinking on the immunology of Graves' disease. Thyroid Today. 1992;**15**:1-11

[18] Laurberg P, Pedersen KM, Vestergaard H, Sigurdsson G. High incidence of multinodular toxic goitre in the elderly population in a low iodine intake area vs. high incidence of Graves' disease in the young in a high iodine intake area: Comparative surveys of thyrotoxicosis epidemiology in East-Jutland Denmark and Iceland. Journal of Internal Medicine. 1991;**229**:415

[19] Radosavljević VR, Janković SM, Marinković JM. Stressful life events in the pathogenesis of Graves' disease. European Journal of Endocrinology. 1996;**134**:699

[20] McDermott MT, Burman KD, Hofeldt FD, Kidd GS. Lithium-associated thyrotoxicosis. The American Journal of Medicine. 1986;**80**:1245

[21] Carella C, Mazziotti G, Amato G, et al. Clinical review 169: Interferon-alpha-related thyroid disease: Pathophysiological, epidemiological, and clinical aspects. The Journal of Clinical Endocrinology & Metabolism. 2004;**89**:3656

[22] Daniels GH, Vladic A, Brinar V, et al. Alemtuzumab-related thyroid dysfunction in a phase 2 trial of patients with relapsing-remitting multiple sclerosis. The Journal of Clinical Endocrinology & Metabolism. 2014;**99**:80

[23] Brent GA. Clinical practice. Graves' disease. The New England Journal of Medicine. 2008;**358**:2594

[24] Fatourechi V, McConahey WM, Woolner LB. Hyperthyroidism associated with histologic Hashimoto's thyroiditis. Mayo Clinic Proceedings. 1971;**46**:682

[25] Rieu M, Richard A, Rosilio M, Laplanche S, Ropion V, Fombeur JP, et al. Effects of thyroid status on thyroid autoimmunity expression in euthyroid and hypothyroid patients with Hashimoto's thyroiditis. Clinical Endocrinology. 1994;**40**:529-535

[26] Rubin RA, Guay AT. Susceptibility to subacute thyroiditis is genetically influenced: Familial occurrence in identical twins. Thyroid. 1991;**1**:157-161

[27] Curtis RE, Rowlings PA, Deeg HJ, Shriner DA, Socie G, Travis LB, et al. Solid cancers after bone marrow transplantation. The New England Journal of Medicine. 1997;**336**:897-904

[28] Pacini F, Vorontsova T, Demidchik EP, Molinaro E, Agate L, Romei C, et al. Post-chernobyl thyroid carcinoma in belarus children and adolescents: Comparison with naturally occurring thyroid carcinoma in Italy and France. The Journal of Clinical Endocrinology & Metabolism. 1997;**82**:3563-3569

[29] Boelaert K, Horacek J, Holder RL, Watkinson JC, Sheppard MC, Franklyn JA. Serum thyrotropin concentration as a novel predictor of malignancy in thyroid nodules investigated by fine-needle aspiration. The Journal of Clinical Endocrinology & Metabolism. 2006;**91**:4295-4301

[30] Haymart MR, Repplinger DJ, Leverson GE, Elson DF, Sippel RS, Jaume JC, et al. Higher serum thyroid stimulating hormone level in thyroid nodule patients is associated with greater risks of differentiated thyroid cancer and advanced tumor stage. The Journal of Clinical Endocrinology & Metabolism. 2008;**93**:809-814

[31] Wanet PM, Sand A, Abramovici J. Physical and clinical evaluation of high-resolution thyroid pinhole tomography. Journal of Nuclear Medicine. 1996;**37**:2017-2020

[32] Gharib H, Papini E. Thyroid nodules: Clinical importance, assessment, and treatment.

Endocrinology and Metabolism Clinics of North America. 2007;**36**:707-735, vi

[33] Lowhagen T, Granberg PO, Lundell G, Skinnari P, Sundblad R, Willems JS. Aspiration biopsy cytology (ABC) in nodules of the thyroid gland suspected to be malignant. Surgical Clinics of North America. 1979;**59**:3-18

[34] Alexander EK, Kennedy GC, Baloch ZW, et al. Preoperative diagnosis of benign thyroid nodules with indeterminate cytology. The New England Journal of Medicine. 2012;**367**:705-715

[35] Miller FN, Netterville JL. Surgical management of thyroid and parathyroid disorders. The Medical Clinics of North America. 1999;**83**:247-259

[36] Colak T, Akca T, Kanik A, Yapici D, Aydin S. Total versus subtotal thyroidectomy for the management of benign multinodular goiter in an endemic region. ANZ Journal of Surgery. 2004;**74**(11):974-978

[37] Cirocchi R, Trastulli S, Randolph J, Guarino S, Di Rocco G, Arezzo A, et al. Total or near-total thyroidectomy versus subtotal thyroidectomy for multinodular non-toxic goitre in adults. Cochrane Database of Systematic Reviews. 2015;**8**:CD010370

[38] Rotondi M, Amato G, Del Buono A, Mazziotti G, Manganella G, Biondi B, et al. Postintervention serum TSH levels may be useful to differentiate patients who should undergo levothyroxine suppressive therapy after thyroid surgery for multinodular goiter in a region with moderate iodine deficiency. Thyroid. 2000;**10**:1081-1085

[39] Hegedus L, Nygaard B, Hansen JM. Is routine thyroxine treatment to hinder postoperative recurrence of nontoxic goiter justified? The Journal of Clinical Endocrinology & Metabolism. 1999;**84**:756-760

[40] Celani MF, Mariani M, Mariani G. On the usefulness of levothyroxine suppressive therapy in the medical treatment of benign solitary, solid or predominantly solid, thyroid nodules. Acta Endocrinologica. 1990;**123**:603-608

[41] Wesche MF, Tiel VBMM, Lips P, Smits NJ, Wiersinga WM. A randomized trial comparing levothyroxine with radioactive iodine in the treatment of sporadic nontoxic goiter. The Journal of Clinical Endocrinology & Metabolism. 2001;**86**:998-1005

[42] Yousef A, Clark J, Suhail AR. Thyroxine suppression therapy for benign, non-functioning solitary thyroid nodules: A quality-effects meta-analysis. Clinical Medicine & Research. 2010;**8**(3-4):150-158

[43] Lima N, Knobel M, Cavaliere H, Sztejnsznajd C, Tomimori E, Medeiros-Neto G. Levothyroxine suppressive therapy is partially effective in treating patients with benign, solid thyroid nodules and multinodular goiters. Thyroid. 1997;**7**(5):691-697

[44] Azizi F, Takyar M, Madreseh E, Amouzegar A. Treatment of toxic multinodular goiter: Comparison of radioiodine and long-term methimazole treatment. Thyroid. 2019;**29**(5):625-630

[45] Kaniuka-Jakubowska S, Lewczuk A, Mizan-Gross K, Piskunowicz M, Zapaśnik A, Lass P, et al. Large multinodular goiter--outpatient radioiodine treatment. Endokrynologia Polska. 2015;**66**(4):301-307

[46] Giusti M, Caorsi V, Mortara L, Caputo M, Monti E, Schiavo M, et al. Long-term outcome after radioiodine therapy with adjuvant rhTSH treatment: Comparison between patients with non-toxic and pre-toxic large multinodulargoitre. Endocrine. 2014;**45**(2):221-229

[47] Giusti M, Cappi C, Santaniello B, Ceresola E, Augeri C, Lagasio C. Safety and efficacy of administering 0.2 mg of recombinant human TSH for two consecutive days as an adjuvant to therapy with low radioiodine doses in elderly out-patients with large nontoxic multinodular goiter. Minerva Endocrinologica. 2006;**31**(3):191-209

[48] Medeiros-Neto G, Knobel M. Iodine deficiency disorders. In: Jameson JL, De Groot LJ, editors. Endocrinology. 6th ed. Philadelphia: WB Saunders Co; 2010

Section 4

Goiter - Acute Complication

Chapter 8

Thyroid Storm: Clinical Manifestation, Pathophysiology, and Treatment

Rahul Pandey, Sanjeev Kumar and Narendra Kotwal

Abstract

Thyroid storm is a rare but life-threatening endocrine emergency. It is an acute exaggerated clinical manifestation of thyrotoxic state. The exact incidence is unknown. It occurs in 1–2% of patients admitted for thyrotoxicosis. It has a mortality of 10–20%. This chapter would help us to understand its clinical manifestations, pathophysiology, and effective treatment. Terminal learning objective would be to diagnose impending storm early and start prompt treatment in day-to-day practice. The chapter would cover pathophysiology including triggers, clinical features including various diagnostic criteria, diagnosis, and treatment of thyroid storm. Indications of surgical treatment in storm will be discussed.

Keywords: thyroid storm, endocrine emergency, thyroid crisis, thyrotoxic storm, thyrotoxic crisis

1. Introduction

Thyroid storm, also known by its synonyms thyroid crisis, thyrotoxic storm, or thyrotoxic crisis, is an extremely rare but life-threatening endocrine emergency. It is an acute exaggerated clinical manifestation of thyrotoxic state [1]. It was first described by Frank Howard Lahey in 1926 as "the crisis of exophthalmic goiter" [2]. Till date, clinicians are puzzled to accurately describe the signs and symptoms of thyroid storm as it involves almost all systems of the body. Accurately diagnosing the condition is very difficult, and groups around have been working to define a clear diagnostic criterion based on universal clinical parameters [3]. Diagnosing the storm early is crucial in order to improve the morbidity and mortality associated with it.

2. Epidemiology

2.1 Incidence

Incidence of thyroid storm is not precisely known. Incidence in general population was reported as 0.57-0.76 per lac per year in USA and 0.20 per lac per year in Japan, whereas incidence in hospitalized patients was 4.8-5.6 per lac per year [4–6]. Hospital data suggest that it occurs in 1–2% of patients admitted for thyrotoxicosis [5]. It occurs more commonly in women and patients with Graves' disease [7]. Autonomous nodules are the culprit in elderly patients [8].

2.2 Mortality

Seventy-five percent of patients hospitalized with thyroid storm die [9]. Overall mortality rate has been reported to be 10–20% [4, 10–12]. Multiple system dysfunction is the commonest cause of death, followed by heart failure [13], respiratory failure [13], and sepsis [3, 14].

3. Pathophysiology of storm

In order to understand the pathophysiology and rationale of treatment for thyroid storm, we need to understand the normal thyroid hormone physiology. Normal thyroid function is under control of feedback mechanisms between the hypothalamus, anterior pituitary and thyroid gland. "Thyrotropin-releasing hormone" (TRH) stimulates anterior pituitary to release "thyroid-stimulating hormone" (TSH), which binds to its receptor on thyroid gland and stimulates the synthesis and secretion of thyroid hormone. The thyroid hormone synthesis is a five-step process comprising of: (a) iodide trapping; (b) organification—oxidation and iodination; (c) coupling; (d) storage; and (e) release. Transport of iodide into the thyroid follicular cell via a sodium-iodide symporter is the first step in hormone synthesis, known as "iodide trapping." Iodide is then "oxidized and organified" by thyroid peroxidase enzyme (TPO). Iodination of tyrosine residues on thyroglobulin (framework protein for thyroid hormone synthesis) is catalyzed by TPO forming thyroxine (T4) and triiodothyronine (T3). Thyroid hormone acts through intranuclear action of T3 with T4 acting more as a "prohormone" [15]. Twenty percent of T3 comes directly from thyroid gland and 80% of circulating T3 comes from peripheral conversion of T4 to T3. The entire process is controlled by a negative feedback loop with peripheral thyroid hormone inhibiting the release and synthesis of TSH and TRH. Majority of the thyroid hormone is protein-bound (>99%) to thyroid-binding globulin (TBG), transthyretin, and albumin [16] making a "circulating storage pool," while unbound or free hormone is available for uptake into the tissues.

Peripheral conversion of T4 to T3 is done by the 5′-deiodinases. The deiodinase D2 is active in euthyroid state whereas in hyperthyroid state deiodinase D1 is more prevalent. The deiodinase D1 is susceptible to inhibition by thionamide and propylthiouracil (PTU). Glucocorticoids and β-blockers inhibit peripheral conversion of T4 to T3. This understanding will help us understand the rationale behind use of various classes of drugs in the treatment of thyroid storm.

Exact pathophysiology of thyroid storm is poorly understood. Several hypotheses have been postulated for the storm, which are as follows:

3.1 Acute increase in release of T4 or T3 from thyroid gland

It is the most important mechanism behind thyroid storm [17]. Acute increase in T4 or T3 hormones is seen after radioiodine therapy, thyroidectomy, discontinuation of antithyroid drugs, and administration of iodinated contrast agents or iodine [18]. Rapid improvements in clinical condition after reduction in T4 or T3 concentration after peritoneal dialysis or plasmapheresis support this theory [19].

3.2 Acute illness causes decrease in protein binding of T4 and T3 in serum resulting in increase of free T4 and T3

Acute illnesses lead to decrease in protein binding of T4 and T3 [20], either due to decrease in production of transthyretin or due to production of inhibitors of T4- and T3-binding protein [21]. They lead to decrease in bound form of T4 and T3, which ultimately leads to relative increase in serum concentration of the hormones, which causes storm [22].

3.3 Role of sympathetic nervous system activation

Many symptoms and signs of thyroid storm mimic those of catecholamine excess, suggesting the role of sympathetic nervous system activation [23]. Dramatic improvement in symptoms following beta blocker administration supports this hypothesis [24].

3.4 Augmentation of cellular responses to thyroid hormone

In patients with condition of hypoxemia, ketoacidosis, lactic acidosis, and infection, there is augmentation of cellular response to thyroid hormone [25]. There is uncoupling of oxidative phosphorylation leading to generation of ATP, which results in excess utilization of substrate, increased oxygen consumption, thermogenesis, and hyperthermia [26]. Excess heat is dissipated by increased sweating and cutaneous vasodilation, the most common symptoms of thyroid storm.

4. Triggers of thyroid storm

The transition from simple thyrotoxicosis to thyrotoxic crisis requires a superimposed insult. Any primary cause of hyperthyroidism can escalate into thyrotoxic crisis. There are triggers that can induce thyroid storm in patients with unrecognized thyrotoxicosis, which includes nonthyroidal surgery, parturition, major trauma, infection, or iodine exposure from radiocontrast dyes or amiodarone [27]. Common and rare triggers are listed in **Table 1**. Infection is the most common precipitant of thyroid storm in the hospitalized patients [3, 17, 27, 28]. There is no identifiable precipitating factor in about 25–43% of patients of storm [29].

Common	Rare
Infection [6]	Vigorous palpation of thyroid gland [30]
Acute medical illness	Subacute thyroiditis [31]
Acute psychosis [32]	Thyroxine overdosage [33]
Nonthyroidal surgery [18]	Aspirin intoxication [34]
Parturition [35]	Hydatidiform mole [36]
Trauma [37]	OP poisoning [38]
Discontinuation of antithyroid drugs [39]	Neurotoxins [40]
After radioactive iodine therapy [41]	Cytotoxic chemotherapy [42]
Post-thyroidectomy [43]	
After high dose of iodine administration [44]	
Iodinated radiographic contrast agents [45]	

Table 1.
Triggers of thyroid storm.

5. Clinical features and diagnosis

The diagnosis of thyroid storm is purely clinical, and if suspected, treatment should be initiated simultaneously without any delay. Clinical picture comprises of an exaggerated feature of hyperthyroidism accompanied by manifestations of multiorgan dysfunction, with the presence of an acute precipitating factor [46]. Symptoms, signs, and clinical features are listed in **Tables 2–4** respectively.

Hyperpyrexia (104–106°F) with diaphoresis is the key presenting feature. High fever induces profuse sweating and leads to insensible fluid losses, which is a differentiating feature between thyroid storm and thyrotoxicosis [1]. Cardiovascular manifestations include palpitations, tachycardia, exercise intolerance, dyspnea on exertion, widened pulse pressure, myocardial ischemia, and atrial fibrillation. Heart rate > 140/min is out of proportion to the underlying illness [47]. The increased cardiac output and tachyarrhythmia may progress to cardiogenic shock [48, 49]. The central nervous system (CNS) manifestations include agitation, delirium, confusion, stupor, obtundation, and coma. CNS involvement is a poor prognostic factor for mortality [3]. Gastrointestinal (GI) symptoms include nausea, vomiting, diarrhea, abdominal pain, intestinal obstruction, and acute hepatic failure [29]. Vomiting and diarrhea add to significant fluid loss. Liver dysfunction and hepatomegaly are due to hepatic congestion and hypoperfusion, or directly due to hyperthyroidism [17]. Jaundice is a poor prognostic indicator [50]. Unusual presentations include acute abdomen, status epilepticus, rhabdomyolysis, hypoglycemia, lactic acidosis, and disseminated intravascular coagulation [51–54].

Various clinical entities that mimic thyroid storm exist, which confounds the existent diagnostic dilemma, namely, peritonitis [55], sepsis/septic shock [56], heat stroke [57], malignant hyperthermia [58], acute pulmonary edema [59], neuroleptic malignant syndrome [60], and serotonin syndrome [61]. The mimics of thyroid storm are listed in **Table 5**.

Hyperactivity, irritability, dysphoria
Heat intolerance and sweating
Palpitations
Fatigue and weakness
Weight loss with increased appetite
Diarrhea
Polyuria
Oligomenorrhea, loss of libido

Table 2.
Symptoms of thyroid storm.

Tachycardia, atrial fibrillation
Tremor
Goiter
Warm, moist skin
Muscle weakness, proximal myopathy
Lid retraction or lag
Gynecomastia
Signs of ophthalmopathy and dermopathy specific for Grave's disease

Table 3.
Signs of thyroid storm.

Abrupt onset
Fever—high grade
Progressively increasing to lethal levels within 24–48 h
Warm skin, flushing, profuse diaphoresis
Goiter and exophthalmos ±
Tachycardia >140 beats/min, atrial fibrillation
Agitation, delirium, psychosis, coma
Diarrhea, nausea, vomiting, pain abdomen, unexplained jaundice

Table 4.
Clinical features of thyroid storm.

Peritonitis
Sepsis/septic shock
Heat stroke
Malignant hyperthermia
Acute pulmonary edema
Neuroleptic malignant syndrome
Serotonin syndrome
Peritonitis

Table 5.
Mimics of thyroid storm.

Burch and Wartofsky's Diagnostic Criteria for Thyroid Storm

Factor	Score
Thermoregulatory dysfunction (temperature ,°F)	
99-99.9	5
100-100.9	10
101-101.9	15
102-102.9	20
103-103.9	25
>=104	30
Central nervous system effects	
Absent	0
Mild	10
Agitation	
Moderate	20
Delirium	
Psychosis	
Extreme lethargy	
Severe	30
Severe	
Coma	
Gastrointestinal-hepatic dysfunction	
Absent	0
Moderate	10
Diarrhea	
Nausea-vomiting	
Abdominal pain	
Severe	20
Unexplained jaundice	

Factor	Score
Cardiovascular dysfunction (tachycardia, beats per minute)	
90-109	5
110-119	10
120-129	15
130-139	20
>=140	25
Congestive heart failure	
Absent	
Mild	0
Pedal edema	5
Moderate	
Bibasilar rales	10
Severe	
Pulmonary edema	15
Atrial fibrillation	
Absent	0
Present	10
Precipitant History	
Negative	0
Positive	10

No storm	<25
Impending storm	25-44
Thyroid storm	45

Figure 1.
Burch and Wartofsky's diagnostic criteria for thyroid storm [28].

Burch and Wartofsky [28] assigned a numerical score to each of the different signs and symptoms of thyroid storm to establish a diagnostic criterion based on the total score calculated as shown in **Figure 1**. Japan Thyroid Association surveyed the incidence of thyroid storm in Japan and formulated population-specific diagnostic criteria based on the presence of the classic organ system manifestations as shown in **Table 6**.

Both Burch and Wartofsky score (BWS) and the Japan Thyroid Association (JTA) guidelines are acceptable. However, in one study, BWS ≥45 was reported to

Prerequisite for diagnosis		
Presence of thyrotoxicosis with elevated levels of free triiodothyronine (FT3) or free thyroxine (FT4)		
Symptoms		
1. Central nervous system (CNS) manifestations: restlessness, delirium, mental aberration/psychosis, somnolence/lethargy, coma (≥1 on the Japan Coma Scale or ≤14 on the Glasgow Coma Scale)		
2. Fever: ≥ 38°C		
3. Tachycardia: ≥130 beats per minute or heart rate ≥ 130 in atrial fibrillation		
4. Congestive heart failure (CHF): pulmonary edema, wet crackles over more than half of the lung field, cardiogenic shock, or Class IV by the New York Heart Association or ≥Class III in the Killip classification		
5. Gastrointestinal (GI)/hepatic manifestations: nausea, vomiting, diarrhea, or a total bilirubin level ≥ 3.0 mg/dL		
Diagnosis		
Grade of thyroid storm (TS)	Combinations of features	Requirements for diagnosis
TS1	First combination	Thyrotoxicosis and at least one CNS manifestation and fever, tachycardia, CHF, or GI/ hepatic manifestations
TS1	Alternate combination	Thyrotoxicosis and at least three combinations of fever, tachycardia, CHF, or GI/ hepatic manifestations
TS2	First combination	Thyrotoxicosis and a combination of two of the following: fever, tachycardia, CHF, or GI/ hepatic manifestations
TS2	Alternate combination	Patients who met the diagnosis of TS1 except that serum FT3 or FT4 level are not available
Exclusion and provisions		
Cases are excluded when clear cut underlying pathology is present for the following symptoms: fever (e.g., pneumonia and malignant hyperthermia), impaired consciousness (e.g., psychiatric disorders and cerebrovascular disease), heart failure (e.g., acute myocardial infarction), and liver disorders (e.g., viral hepatitis and acute liver failure). Therefore, it is difficult to determine whether the symptom is caused by TS or is simply a manifestation of an underlying disease; the symptom should be regarded as being due to a TS that is caused by these precipitating factors. Clinical judgment in this matter is required.		

TS1, "Definite" TS; TS2, "Suspected" TS.
Adapted from: Akamizu et al. [3].

Table 6.
The diagnostic criteria for thyroid storm (TS) of the Japan Thyroid Association.

be more sensitive than JTA guidelines in detecting patients with storm [62, 63]. It is recommended to use both criteria to increase the accuracy of the diagnosis of thyroid storm [44, 63].

Although diagnosis of thyroid storm is clinical, laboratory values aid in the diagnosis and treatment. A complete workup including estimation of TSH, free T4, and free T3 should be done in the intensive care unit (ICU) setting. Leukocytosis indicates infection (commonest factor for storm). Elevated blood urea nitrogen [3] and liver function abnormalities with elevation in the transaminases and hyperbilirubinemia indicate irreversible abnormalities. Hypercalcemia may be found due to the high bone resorption that accompanies hyperthyroidism and can exacerbate dehydration. Hyperglycemia is due to a combination of increased catecholamine inhibition of insulin release and increased gluconeogenesis [64].

6. Management

The treatment of thyroid storm should be initiated as soon as the diagnosis is suspected. Patients should be triaged to an intensive care setting for close monitoring and aggressive treatment. A multidisciplinary team approach is important in order to successfully offer the patient all possible therapeutic options. Immediate goals of thyroid-specific therapy should be targeted to decrease thyroid hormone synthesis and release, decrease peripheral action of thyroid hormone, and treat the precipitating cause.

6.1 Inhibiting new thyroid hormone synthesis

The first-line therapy in treating thyroid storm consists of inhibiting new thyroid hormone production. This approach most commonly utilizes thionamides which includes thiouracils (PTU) and imidazoles (methimazole and carbimazole). They inhibit thyroid peroxidase (TPO), thereby inhibiting formation of T3 and T4 from thyroglobulin [65]. Both methimazole and PTU are used but PTU is favored during thyroid storm due to its additional benefit over carbimazole and methimazole, namely rapid onset of action and inhibition of peripheral conversion of T4 to T3 mediated by peripheral deiodinase. In addition, PTU can be safely used in pregnancy.

The dose of PTU is 600–1500 mg/day in divided doses every 4–6 h [27, 28, 66] with a loading dose of 600 mg. Dose of methimazole is 80–120 mg daily in divided doses every 4–6 h [27, 28, 66]. The American Association of Clinical Endocrinologist/ American Thyroid Association guidelines recommend 500–1000 mg loading dose of PTU followed by 250 mg every 4 h and 60–80 mg/day of methimazole in divided doses [67]. Routes of administration include intravenous, enteral, and per rectal as suppository or retention enema. PTU is relatively insoluble at physiologic pH, therefore its intravenous preparation and administration are difficult. Intravenous methimazole can be prepared easily by dissolving methimazole powder in normal saline [68].

Nonradioactive iodine also decreases new thyroid hormone synthesis. It is due to the inhibition of organic binding of iodide to thyroglobulin as plasma iodide levels reach a critical threshold, a phenomenon known as the Wolff-Chaikoff effect. The effect is transient, lasting for about 50 h, as the thyroid eventually escapes/ adapts to prolonged iodide excess [69]. Inorganic iodine may be given orally as a saturated solution of potassium iodide (SSKI) by administering five drops (0.25 mL or 250 mg) every 6 h or as Lugol's solution (eight drops given every 6 h) [28, 67]. Routes can be enteral, rectal, or intravenous. SSKI is prepared for rectal dosing by mixing 1 g of iodide in 60 mL of water and administering 2 g/day in divided doses [70]. Lugol's solution can be given rectally in doses of 4 mL (80 drops) per day [71]. Iodine should be given at least 30 min after administering thionamides to avoid the iodine serving as a substrate for new thyroid hormone production and worsening the hyperthyroidism. Thionamides must be continued during therapy with iodine to avoid organification of iodine and increased thyroid hormone production. Iodine administration delays definitive treatment of patients' hyperthyroidism with radioactive iodine [27, 28]. Therefore, iodine should be used only when the end goal is thyroidectomy.

Lithium hampers T4 and T3 synthesis by inhibiting the coupling of iodotyrosine residues. When iodine administration is not possible (secondary to iodine induced anaphylaxis) or desired, lithium may be substituted. It is administered at doses of 300 mg every 6–8 h with monitoring of serum levels.

6.2 Inhibiting thyroid hormone release

The next line of treatment is inhibiting the release of preformed hormone. Iodine administration, additionally, blocks the release of preformed hormone by inhibiting the release of iodothyronines (T3 and T4) from thyroglobulin [28, 72]. This effect of iodine has a faster onset than PTU, which blocks synthesis in a thyroid gland that has a large store of already formed hormone [73]. The combination therapy of thionamides and iodine decrease serum T4 levels to normal range in 4–5 days [74].

6.3 Inhibiting the peripheral effect of thyroid hormone

Both α- and β-adrenergic stimulation are enhanced in thyroid storm. Thus, adrenergic blockade is an integral part of the treatment. β-Blockers have been used in treatment of both uncomplicated and complicated hyperthyroidism [75]. Propranolol is the most commonly used β-blocker due to its nonselective β-adrenergic antagonism and its ability to block the peripheral conversion of T4 to T3. The recommended dose is 60–120 mg orally every 6 h [64]. For a more rapid effect, intravenous propranolol or a shorter acting β-blocker such as esmolol can be used. The dose of intravenous propranolol is 0.5–1.0 mg slow infusion for an initial dose and then 1–2 mg at 15-min intervals while monitoring the heart rate carefully. Esmolol is given as an initial bolus of 0.25–0.5 mg/kg followed by a continuous infusion rate of 0.05–0.1 mg/kg per minute [73].

6.4 Inhibiting enterohepatic circulation of thyroid hormone

Enterohepatic circulation of thyroid hormone is targeted for severe and refractory thyroid storm. Thyroid hormone is metabolized in the liver where it is conjugated to glucuronides and sulfates. Conjugated products are excreted into the intestine through bile, where free hormones are released, reabsorbed, and circulated. This is enterohepatic circulation of thyroid hormone. Cholestyramine binds the conjugation products and promotes their excretion, and can be used to decrease thyroid hormone levels. The recommended dose is 1–4 g twice a day [76–78].

6.5 Other therapies

The oral iodinated contrast agents are inhibitors of both deiodinases D1 and D2 and help in lowering T3 levels. Additionally, they inhibit new thyroid hormone synthesis and release of preformed hormones from the gland. They are given as 2 g loading dose followed by 1 g daily [74, 79]. Lower doses are given for preoperative preparation for thyroid surgery [80, 81] and as an adjunct to thionamides in treatment of Graves' disease [82].

6.6 Supportive and resuscitative measures

Resuscitative measures should be initiated immediately in an ICU setting. Urgent addressal of systemic decompensation requires correction of hyperthermia, dehydration, congestive heart failure, dysrhythmia, and prevention of adrenal crisis [73]. Hyperthermia should be controlled with peripheral cooling and antipyretics. Acetaminophen is preferred over salicylates as salicylates increase free hormone levels by decreasing binding to T4-binding globulin, thereby exacerbating thyroid storm [83]. The peripheral cooling should be done with ice packs, cooling blankets, or alcohol sponges. Fluid loss due to hyperpyrexia, diarrhea, and vomiting should be corrected immediately.

The hypothalamo-pituitary-adrenal axis is impaired in thyrotoxicosis with a decrease in adrenal reserve. Despite increased production of cortisol by the adrenal gland to compensate for accelerated glucocorticosteroid metabolism in hyperthyroid states, a subnormal response of the adrenal glands to adrenocortico-stimulating hormone occurs. Corticosteroids are therefore used as adjunct therapy in thyroid storm to prevent adrenal insufficiency. It also helps in decreasing the peripheral conversion of T4 to T3 [84]. A loading dose of 300 mg of hydrocortisone intravenously followed by 100 mg every 8 h is recommended [67].

The treatment of thyroid storm is not complete and effective until correctable precipitating factors are addressed (**Table 1**). Any focus of infection should be thoroughly investigated and proper antibiotics should be started based on sensitivity. In addition, any metabolic abnormalities, such as diabetic ketoacidosis, stroke, or pulmonary emboli, should be treated as per standard protocols.

6.7 Therapeutic plasma exchange

In refractory cases of thyrotoxic crisis with no clinical improvement alternative measures to clear thyroid hormone from the circulation should be instituted. Therapeutic plasma exchange (TPE) is effective in rapidly reducing thyroid hormone levels [85]. The patient's plasma is extracted from the components of blood, and replaced with albumin or fresh frozen plasma [85, 86]. TBG with bound thyroid hormone is removed from circulation, and the colloid replacement (usually albumin) provides unsaturated binding sites for circulating free thyroid hormone. Various techniques of exchange transfusion have evolved since its first description in 1970 by Ashkar et al. [87]. Plasma exchange, single pass albumin dialysis, and charcoal hemoperfusion have all demonstrated a reduction in free T3 and free T4 levels [85].

TPE is an option when clinical deterioration in thyroid storm occurs despite the use of first- and second-line therapies. Muller et al. suggested early initiation of TPE with the following indications: severe symptoms (cardio-thyrotoxicosis, neurologic manifestations, and severe myopathy); rapid clinical deterioration; contraindications to other therapies; and failure of conventional therapeutics [88]. The American Society for Apheresis (ASFA) recommends that TPE be performed at a frequency of daily to every 2–3 days until clinical improvement is noted. Complications of TPE are seen in 5% of patients and include hypotension, hemolysis, allergic reactions, coagulopathy, vascular injury, and infection [86, 88, 89].

Absolute indication	Relative indication
Failed medical therapy	Symptomatic goiter
Severe reaction to antithyroid drugs	Pregnancy
Not a candidate for radio ablation therapy	Severe Grave's ophthalmopathy
Persistent thyrotoxicosis despite maximum antithyroid drug/radio ablation therapy Underlying thyroid carcinoma Suspicious/malignant nodules on FNAC	Refractory thyroiditis Amiodarone related Toxic adenoma

Table 7.
Indications of surgery.

6.8 Surgical management

Achieving a euthyroid state is first and foremost requisite prior to surgical management using the above-mentioned medical treatment strategies [27]. However, there is a subset of patients who fail medical management despite all of the most aggressive treatment modalities. This occurs more commonly in iodine-deficient areas, where thyroid storm is mostly related to iodine contamination in patients with thyroid autonomy. These patients are particularly resistant to even high-dose thionamides or iodine therapy because of the large intrathyroidal iodine pool [90]. The broad indications of surgery have been listed in **Table** 7.

All measures should be employed to stabilize the patient prior to considering emergent surgical management. Surgical team should be involved early (within 12–72 h) if the patient is not responding to medical therapy. The surgical options involve a subtotal or near-total thyroidectomy [73]. The surgery produces rapid resolution of the hyperthyroidism as very little thyroid tissue remains. This allows cessation of the thionamides soon after the surgery. Corticosteroid and β-blocker should be continued perioperatively and slowly weaned off over the ensuing weeks [27].

6.9 Newer agents

Biological agent Rituximab (anti-CD20 monoclonal antibody which depletes B lymphocytes) and various other emerging therapies have shown promise in the treatment of Graves' ophthalmopathy, but the role of these agents in the management of the thyrotoxic state is less clear [17, 91–93].

7. Conclusion

Thyroid storm is an endocrine emergency that is associated with high morbidity and mortality if not promptly recognized and treated. Multidisciplinary treatment

Block synthesis (anti thyroid drugs)
Block release (iodine)
Block T4 to T3 conversion (high dose PTU, propranolol, corticosteroid)
Beta blocker
Block enterohepatic circulation (cholestyramine)

Table 8.
Five B's of thyroid storm.

in an intensive care setting is usually needed. Treatment involves addressing all steps of thyroid hormone synthesis, release, and action, in a well-defined order, while providing supportive care. Remember five B's in thyroid storm as listed in **Table 8**. Treating precipitating factors is an integral part of the management.

Conflict of interest

The authors declare no conflict of interest.

Author details

Rahul Pandey*, Sanjeev Kumar and Narendra Kotwal
Armed Forces Clinic, New Delhi, India

*Address all correspondence to: rahuladviksimpy@gmail.com

References

[1] Leung AM. Thyroid Emergencies. PubMed-NCBI [Internet]. Available from: https://www.ncbi.nlm.nih.gov/pubmed/27598067

[2] Lahey FH. Apathetic thyroidism. Annals of Surgery. 1931;**93**(5):1026-1030

[3] Akamizu T, Satoh T, Isozaki O, Suzuki A, Wakino S, Iburi T, et al. Diagnostic criteria, clinical features, and incidence of thyroid storm based on nationwide surveys. Thyroid. 2012;**22**(7):661-679

[4] Diagnostic criteria, clinical features, and incidence of thyroid storm based on nationwide surveys. PubMed-NCBI [Internet]. Available from: https://www.ncbi.nlm.nih.gov/pubmed?term=22690898

[5] National Trends in Incidence, Mortality, and Clinical Outcomes of Patients Hospitalized for Thyrotoxicosis With and Without Thyroid Storm in the Un. PubMed-NCBI [Internet]. Available from: https://www.ncbi.nlm.nih.gov/pubmed?term=30382003

[6] Akamizu T. Thyroid storm: A Japanese perspective. Thyroid. 2018;**28**(1):32-40

[7] Bartalena L. Graves' disease: Complications. In: Feingold KR, Anawalt B, Boyce A, Chrousos G, Dungan K, Grossman A, et al., editors. Endotext. South Dartmouth (MA): MDText.com, Inc.; 2000. Available from: http://www.ncbi.nlm.nih.gov/books/NBK285551/

[8] Holzheimer RG. Benign nodular thyroid disease [Internet]. Zuckschwerdt; 2001. Available from: https://www.ncbi.nlm.nih.gov/books/NBK6893/

[9] Dillmann WH. Thyroid storm. Current Therapy in Endocrinology and Metabolism. 1997;**6**:81-85

[10] Clinical characteristics and outcome of thyroid storm: a case series and review of neuropsychiatric derangements in thyrotoxicosis. PubMed-NCBI [Internet]. [cited: 25 July 2019]. Available from: https://www.ncbi.nlm.nih.gov/pubmed?term=25370315

[11] Clinical features and hospital outcomes in thyroid storm: A retrospective cohort study. PubMed-NCBI [Internet]. Available from: https://www.ncbi.nlm.nih.gov/pubmed?term=25343237

[12] Factors associated with mortality of thyroid storm: Analysis using a national inpatient database in Japan. PubMed-NCBI [Internet]. Available from: https://www.ncbi.nlm.nih.gov/pubmed?term=26886648

[13] Nai Q, Ansari M, Pak S, Tian Y, Amzad-Hossain M, Zhang Y, et al. Cardiorespiratory failure in thyroid storm: Case report and literature review. Journal of Clinical Medical Research. 2018;**10**(4):351-357

[14] Feldt-Rasmussen U, Emerson CH. Further thoughts on the diagnosis and diagnostic criteria for thyroid storm. Thyroid. 2012;**22**(11):1094-1095

[15] Brent GA. Mechanisms of thyroid hormone action. The Journal of Clinical Investigation. 2012;**122**(9):3035-3043

[16] Refetoff S. Thyroid hormone serum transport proteins. In: Feingold KR, Anawalt B, Boyce A, Chrousos G, Dungan K, Grossman A, et al., editors. Endotext. South Dartmouth (MA): MDText.com, Inc.; 2000 Available from: http://www.ncbi.nlm.nih.gov/books/NBK285566/

[17] Carroll R, Matfin G. Endocrine and metabolic emergencies: Thyroid storm. Therapeutic Advances in Endocrinology and Metabolism. 2010;**1**(3):139-145

[18] Idrose AM. Acute and emergency care for thyrotoxicosis and thyroid storm. Acute Medicine & Surgery. 2015;**2**(3):147-157

[19] Carhill A, Gutierrez A, Lakhia R, Nalini R. Surviving the storm: Two cases of thyroid storm successfully treated with plasmapheresis. BMJ Case Reports. 2012;**2012**:bcr2012006696

[20] Tibaldi JM, Surks MI. Effects of nonthyroidal illness on thyroid function. The Medical Clinics of North America. 1985;**69**(5):899-911

[21] Schussler GC. The thyroxine-binding proteins. Thyroid. 2000;**10**(2):141-149

[22] Malik R, Hodgson H. The relationship between the thyroid gland and the liver. QJM: An International Journal of Medicine. 2002;**95**(9):559-569

[23] Parsons V, Ramsay I. Thyroid and adrenal relationships. Postgraduate Medical Journal. 1968;**44**(511):377-384

[24] Tjokroprawiro A. Review Article and Clinical Experience: Graves' Disease and Thyroid Storm ATD Therapy, Formulas TS-41668, CS-7.3.7. In 2007

[25] Pangtey GS, Baruah U, Baruah MP, Bhagat S. Thyroid emergencies: New insight into old problems. The Journal of the Association of Physicians of India. 2017;**65**(8):68-76

[26] Ricquier D, Bouillaud F. Mitochondrial uncoupling proteins: From mitochondria to the regulation of energy balance. The Journal of Physiology. 2000;**529**(Pt 1):3-10

[27] Nayak B, Burman K. Thyrotoxicosis and thyroid storm. Endocrinology and Metabolism Clinics of North America. 2006;**35**(4):663-686 vii

[28] Burch HB, Wartofsky L. Life-threatening thyrotoxicosis. Thyroid storm. Endocrinology and Metabolism Clinics of North America. 1993;**22**(2):263-277

[29] Wartofsky L, Klubo-Gwiezdzinska J. Thyroid storm (thyrotoxic crisis). In: Luster M, Duntas LH, Wartofsky L, editors. The Thyroid and Its Diseases: A Comprehensive Guide for the Clinician. Cham: Springer International Publishing; 2019. pp. 357-366. DOI: 10.1007/978-3-319-72102-6_25

[30] Yatavelli RK, Levine SN. Transient hyperthyroidism induced by thyroid ultrasound. The Annals of Otology, Rhinology, and Laryngology. 2018;**127**(8):558-562

[31] Salih AM, Kakamad FH, Rawezh QS, Masrur SA, Shvan HM, Hawbash MR, et al. Subacute thyroiditis causing thyrotoxic crisis; A case report with literature review. International Journal of Surgery Case Reports. 2017;**33**:112-114

[32] Irwin R, Ellis PM, Delahunt J. Psychosis following acute alteration of thyroid status. The Australian and New Zealand Journal of Psychiatry. 1997;**31**(5):762-764

[33] Medeiros-Neto G. Thyroxine poisoning. In: Feingold KR, Anawalt B, Boyce A, Chrousos G, Dungan K, Grossman A, et al., editors. Endotext. South Dartmouth (MA): MDText.com, Inc.; 2000. Available from: http://www.ncbi.nlm.nih.gov/books/NBK279036/

[34] Sebe A, Satar S, Sari A. Thyroid storm induced by aspirin intoxication and the effect of hemodialysis: A case report. Advances in Therapy. 2004;**21**(3):173-177

[35] Ma Y, Li H, Liu J, Lin X, Liu H. Impending thyroid storm in a pregnant woman with undiagnosed hyperthyroidism. Medicine. 2018;**97**(3). Available from: https://www.ncbi.nlm.nih.gov/pmc/articles/PMC5779755/

[36] Moskovitz JB, Bond MC. Molar pregnancy-induced thyroid storm. The Journal of Emergency Medicine. 2010;**38**(5):e71-e76

[37] Karaören GY, Sahin OT, Erbesler ZA, Bakan N. Thyroid storm due to head injury. Ulus Travma Acil Cerrahi Derg [Turkish Journal of Trauma and Emergency Surgery]. 2014;**20**(4):305-307

[38] Yuan Y-D, Seak C-J, Lin C-C, Lin L-J. Thyroid storm precipitated by organophosphate intoxication. American Journal of Emergency Medicine. 2007;**25**(7):861.e1-861.e3

[39] Liu J, Fu J, Xu Y, Wang G. Antithyroid drug therapy for Graves' disease and implications for recurrence. International Journal of Endocrinology. 2017;**2017** Available from: https://www.ncbi.nlm.nih.gov/pmc/articles/PMC5424485/

[40] Dolan LC, Matulka RA, Burdock GA. Naturally occurring food toxins. Toxins. 2010;**2**(9):2289-2332

[41] Vennard K, Gilbert MP. Thyroid storm and complete heart block after treatment with radioactive iodine. Case Reports in Endocrinology. 2018 Available from: https://www.hindawi.com/journals/crie/2018/8214169/ref/

[42] Al-Anazi KA, Inam S, Jeha MT, Judzewitch R. Thyrotoxic crisis induced by cytotoxic chemotherapy. Supportive Care in Cancer. 2005;**13**(3):196-198

[43] Toft AD, Irvine WJ, Sinclair I, McIntosh D, Seth J, Cameron EHD. Thyroid function after surgical treatment of thyrotoxicosis. The New England Journal of Medicine. 1978;**298**(12):643-647

[44] Ross DS, Burch HB, Cooper DS, Greenlee MC, Laurberg P, Maia AL, et al. 2016 American Thyroid Association guidelines for diagnosis and management of hyperthyroidism and other causes of thyrotoxicosis. Thyroid. 2016;**26**(10):1343-1421

[45] Thomsen HS. European Society of Urogenital Radiology (ESUR) guidelines on the safe use of iodinated contrast media. European Journal of Radiology. 2006;**60**(3):307-313

[46] Wartofsky L. Clinical criteria for the diagnosis of thyroid storm. Thyroid. Available from: https://www.liebertpub.com/doi/10.1089/thy.2012.2207.ed1

[47] Klein I, Danzi S. Thyroid disease and the heart. Circulation. 2007;**116**(15):1725-1735

[48] Klein I, Ojamaa K. Thyroid hormone and the cardiovascular system. The New England Journal of Medicine. 2001;**344**(7):501-509

[49] Ngo SYA, Chew HC. When the storm passes unnoticed—A case series of thyroid storm. Resuscitation. 2007;**73**(3):485-490

[50] Choudhary AM, Roberts I. Thyroid storm presenting with liver failure. Journal of Clinical Gastroenterology. 1999;**29**(4):318-321

[51] Harwood-Nuss AL, Martel TJ. An unusual cause of abdominal pain in a young woman. Annals of Emergency Medicine. 1991;**20**(5):574-582

[52] Deng Y, Zheng W, Zhu J. Successful treatment of thyroid crisis accompanied by hypoglycemia, lactic acidosis, and multiple organ failure. American Journal of Emergency Medicine. 2012;**30**(9):2094.e5-2094.e6

[53] Lee TG, Ha CK, Lim BH. Thyroid storm presenting as status epilepticus and stroke. Postgraduate Medical Journal. 1997;**73**(855):61-61

[54] Summachiwakij S, Sachmechi I. Rhabdomyolysis induced by

nonstrenuous exercise in a patient with graves' disease. Case Reports in Endocrinology. 2014;**2014**:286450-286450

[55] Shah SR, Millan T, Alamzaib SM, Luu S-W. Idiopathic thyroid storm mimicking SIRS in a patient with hypothyroidism—A diagnostic dilemma. Journal of Community Hospital Internal Medicine Perspectives. 2018;**8**(6):368-369

[56] Rayner SG, Hosseini F, Adedipe AA. Sepsis mimicking thyroid storm in a patient with methimazole-induced agranulocytosis. BMJ Case Reports. 2013;**2013**:bcr2013200145

[57] Mørch SS, Andersen JDH, Bestle MH. Heat stroke: A medical emergency appearing in new regions. Case Reports in Critical Care. 2017;**2017**:6219236-6219236

[58] Kiranchand N, Mallanna B, Bhaskar SB, Srinivasalu D. Suspected malignant hyperthermia in a patient undergoing thyroidectomy. Indian Journal of Anaesthesia. 2013;**57**(2):209-210

[59] Chong HW, See KC, Phua J. Thyroid storm with multiorgan failure. Thyroid. 2010;**20**(3):333-336

[60] Ioos V, Das V, Maury E, Baudel J-L, Guéchot J, Guidet B, et al. A thyrotoxicosis outbreak due to dietary pills in Paris. Therapeutics and Clinical Risk Management. 2008;**4**(6):1375

[61] Ronan GP, Ronan N, McGettigan S, Browne G. Serotonin syndrome unmasking thyrotoxicosis. BML Case Reports. 2019;**12**(3):e228404

[62] Angell TE, Lechner MG, Nguyen CT, Salvato VL, Nicoloff JT, LoPresti JS. Clinical features and hospital outcomes in thyroid storm: A retrospective cohort study. The Journal of Clinical Endocrinology and Metabolism. 2015;**100**(2):451-459

[63] Satoh T, Isozaki O, Suzuki A, Wakino S, Iburi T, Tsuboi K, et al. 2016 guidelines for the management of thyroid storm from the Japan Thyroid association and Japan Endocrine Society (first edition). Endocrine Journal. 2016;**63**(12):1025-1064

[64] Stathatos N, Wartofsky L. Thyrotoxic storm. Journal of Intensive Care Medicine. 2002;**17**(1):1-7

[65] Davies T, Larsen P. Thyrotoxicosis. In: Willams Textbook of Endocrinology. 11th ed. Philadelphia, PA: Saunders Elsevier; 2007. pp. 333-375

[66] Cooper DS. Antithyroid drugs. The New England Journal of Medicine. 2005;**352**(9):905-917

[67] Bahn RS, Burch HB, Cooper DS, Garber JR, Greenlee MC, Klein I, et al. Hyperthyroidism and other causes of thyrotoxicosis: Management guidelines of the American Thyroid Association and American Association of Clinical Endocrinologists. Thyroid. 2011;**17**(3):456-520

[68] Hodak SP, Huang C, Clarke D, Burman KD, Jonklaas J, Janicic-Kharic N. Intravenous methimazole in the treatment of refractory hyperthyroidism. Thyroid. 2006;**16**(7):691-695

[69] Eng PH, Cardona GR, Fang SL, Previti M, Alex S, Carrasco N, et al. Escape from the acute Wolff-Chaikoff effect is associated with a decrease in thyroid sodium/iodide symporter messenger ribonucleic acid and protein. Endocrinology. 1999;**140**(8):3404-3410

[70] Yeung SC, Go R, Balasubramanyam A. Rectal administration of iodide and propylthiouracil in the treatment of thyroid storm. Thyroid. 1995;**5**(5):403-405

[71] Ogiso S, Inamoto S, Hata H, Yamaguchi T, Otani T, Koizumi K. Successful treatment of gastric

perforation with thyrotoxic crisis. American Journal of Emergency Medicine. 2008;**26**(9):1065.e3-1065.e4

[72] Woeber KA. Iodine and thyroid disease. The Medical Clinics of North America. 1991;**75**(1):169-178

[73] Sosa JA. Textbook of endocrine surgery, 2nd edition. Annals of Surgery. 2006;**244**(2):322-322

[74] Wartofsky L, Ransil BJ, Ingbar SH. Inhibition by iodine of the release of thyroxine from the thyroid glands of patients with thyrotoxicosis. The Journal of Clinical Investigation. 1970;**49**(1):78-86

[75] Hughes G. Management of thyrotoxic crises with a beta-adrenergic blocking agent (Pronethalol). The British Journal of Clinical Practice. 1966;**20**(11):579-581

[76] Mercado M, Mendoza-Zubieta V, Bautista-Osorio R, Espinoza-de los Monteros AL. Treatment of hyperthyroidism with a combination of methimazole and cholestyramine. The Journal of Clinical Endocrinology and Metabolism. 1996;**81**(9):3191-3193

[77] Tsai W-C, Pei D, Wang T-F, Wu D-A, Li J-C, Wei CL, et al. The effect of combination therapy with propylthiouracil and cholestyramine in the treatment of Graves' hyperthyroidism. Clinical Endocrinology. 2005;**62**(5):521-524

[78] Kaykhaei MA, Shams M, Sadegholvad A, Dabbaghmanesh MH, Omrani GR. Low doses of cholestyramine in the treatment of hyperthyroidism. Endocrine. 2008;**34**(1-3):52-55

[79] Papi G, Corsello SM, Pontecorvi A. Clinical concepts on thyroid emergencies. Frontiers in Endocrinology. 2014;**5**:102-102

[80] Langley RW, Burch HB. Perioperative management of the thyrotoxic patient. Endocrinology and Metabolism Clinics of North America. 2003;**32**(2):519-534

[81] Panzer C, Beazley R, Braverman L. Rapid preoperative preparation for severe hyperthyroid graves' disease. The Journal of Clinical Endocrinology and Metabolism. 2004;**89**(5):2142-2144

[82] Roti E, Robuschi G, Gardini E, Montermini M, Salvi M, Manfredi A, et al. Comparison of methimazole, methimazole and sodium ipodate, and methimazole and saturated solution of potassium iodide in the early treatment of hyperthyroid Graves'disease. Clinical Endocrinology. 1988;**28**(3):305-314

[83] Wang R, Nelson JC, Wilcox RB. Salsalate and salicylate binding to and their displacement of thyroxine from thyroxine-binding globulin, transthyrin, and albumin. Thyroid. 1999;**9**(4):359-364

[84] Tsatsoulis A, Johnson EO, Kalogera CH, Seferiadis K, Tsolas O. The effect of thyrotoxicosis on adrenocortical reserve. European Journal of Endocrinology. 2000;**142**(3):231-235

[85] Szczepiorkowski ZM, Winters JL, Bandarenko N, Kim HC, Linenberger ML, Marques MB, et al. Guidelines on the use of therapeutic apheresis in clinical practice—Evidence-based approach from the apheresis applications Committee of the American Society for apheresis. Journal of Clinical Apheresis. 2010;**25**(3):83-177

[86] Ezer A, Caliskan K, Parlakgumus A, Belli S, Kozanoglu I, Yildirim S. Preoperative therapeutic plasma exchange in patients with thyrotoxicosis. Journal of Clinical Apheresis. 2009;**24**(3):111-114

[87] Ashkar FS, Katims RB, Smoak WM, Gilson AJ. Thyroid storm treatment with blood exchange and plasmapheresis. Journal of the American Medical Association. 1970;**214**(7):1275-1279

[88] Muller C, Perrin P, Faller B, Richter S, Chantrel F. Role of plasma exchange in the thyroid storm. Therapeutic Apheresis and Dialysis. 2011;**15**(6):522-531

[89] Chen J-H, Yeh J-H, Lai H-W, Liao C-S. Therapeutic plasma exchange in patients with hyperlipidemic pancreatitis. World Journal of Gastroenterology. 2004;**10**(15):2272-2274

[90] Scholz GH, Hagemann E, Arkenau C, Engelmann L, Lamesch P, Schreiter D, et al. Is there a place for thyroidectomy in older patients with thyrotoxic storm and cardiorespiratory failure? Thyroid. 2003;**13**(10):933-940

[91] Abraham P, Acharya S. Current and emerging treatment options for Graves' hyperthyroidism. Therapeutics and Clinical Risk Management. 2010;**6**:29-40

[92] Bahn RS. Graves' ophthalmopathy. The New England Journal of Medicine. 2010;**362**(8):726-738

[93] Roizen M, Becker CE. Thyroid storm. A review of cases at University of California, San Francisco. California Medicine. 1971;**115**(4):5-9